METHODS IN PHARMACOLOGY AND TOXICOLOGY

Series Editor
Y. James Kang
University of Louisville
School of Medicine
Prospect, Kentucky, USA

For further volumes:
http://www.springer.com/series/7653

Epigenetics and Gene Expression in Cancer, Inflammatory and Immune Diseases

Edited by

Barbara Stefanska

Department of Nutrition Science, Purdue University, West Lafayette, IN, USA

David J. MacEwan

*Department of Molecular and Clinical Pharmacology,
Institute of Translational Medicine, University of Liverpool, Liverpool, UK*

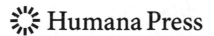
Humana Press

Editors
Barbara Stefanska
Department of Nutrition Science
Purdue University
West Lafayette, IN, USA

David J. MacEwan
Department of Molecular
  and Clinical Pharmacology
Institute of Translational Medicine
University of Liverpool
Liverpool, UK

ISSN 1557-2153   ISSN 1940-6053   (electronic)
Methods in Pharmacology and Toxicology
ISBN 978-1-4939-8289-9   ISBN 978-1-4939-6743-8   (eBook)
DOI 10.1007/978-1-4939-6743-8

Printed on acid-free paper

This Humana Press imprint is published by Springer Nature
The registered company is Springer Science+Business Media LLC
The registered company address is: 233 Spring Street, New York, NY 10013, U.S.A.

Preface

Epigenetics refers to alterations in gene expression without changes in the underlying DNA sequence and consists of three main components: DNA methylation, histone covalent modifications, and noncoding RNA mechanisms. Aberrant epigenetic patterns have been linked to chronic inflammation in numerous studies, which consequently leads to the development of many diseases including cancer, diabetes, multiple sclerosis and other autoimmune diseases, psychiatric, and neurodegenerative disorders. Due to the inherent reversibility of epigenetic states, epigenetic modifications constitute an excellent target for prevention and treatment of these various illnesses. The last two decades of scientific efforts brought about a remarkable move forward in understanding epigenetics in human disease and health, which was made possible with novel advanced methodologies. One of the milestones was introducing genome-wide approaches to studying epigenetics which opened a new emerging field of epigenomics that is useful to a wide range of researchers in different areas.

The vision for *Epigenetics and Gene Expression in Cancer, Inflammatory and Immune Diseases* is to provide pharmacologists, molecular biologists, bioinformaticians, and toxicologists with a background on epigenetics and state-of-the-art techniques in epigenomics. Although the focus of the book is cancer, inflammatory and autoimmune disorders, the presented methodologies can find applications in areas outside of these fields. Chapters discuss three main components of the epigenome and their role in the regulation of gene expression and present a detailed method section specific to studying each component, including data analyses, troubleshooting, and feasibility in different experimental settings. The main topics are high-throughput and targeted methods for DNA methylation analysis, nucleosome position mapping, studying epigenetic effects of gut microbiota, optical imaging for detection of epigenetic aberrations in living cells, methods for microRNA, and histone code profiling.

The book begins with three chapters detailing the methods for DNA methylation profiling. Genome-wide approaches include methylated DNA immunoprecipitation (MeDIP) paired with microarray technology or next generation sequencing, Infinium HumanMethylation450 BeadChip (Illumina 450K), and Reduced Representation Bisulfite Sequencing (RRBS). The protocols are compared and advantages and disadvantages of each are discussed in Chap. 1. RRBS and Illumina 450K are both bisulfite-based methods that measure site-specific methylation, whereas MeDIP-seq and MeDIP-ChIP are enrichment-based methods that provide information on the relative abundance of DNA methylation. Thus, they differ with regard to coverage, sample size, resolution, and discrimination toward CpG rich and CpG poor regions. One must consider which method best suits a particular study in order to generate robust and accurate data. Given the heterogeneity in cell populations, which is of special interest in neuroscience, development of single-cell techniques exploring the epigenome is of high interest. As RRBS requires low starting input DNA, this approach can be applied to single-cell analysis of DNA methylation patterns. Chapter 2 discusses the current issue of cell population heterogeneity in epigenetic profiling and describes how dividing cells into their distinct subpopulations using fluorescence-activated cell sorting (FACS) can help to address this problem. Genome-wide experimental approaches in DNA methylation profiling lead to the discovery of specific CpG sites, regions, and genes that may play a functional role and require further validation with targeted DNA methylation analysis methods. Chapter 3 describes and compares pyrosequencing, quantitative methylated DNA immunoprecipitation (qMeDIP), and methylation-sensitive high-resolution melting (MS-HRM) analysis. These methods replace nowadays bisulfite standard sequencing that is time-consuming, labor intensive, and often underpowered. While pyrosequencing quantitatively measures the percentage of methylation at single CpG resolution, qMeDIP and MS-HRM provide semi-quantitative results often at the region-based resolution.

Components of the epigenome exert effects over each other and participate in the formation of specific patterns of chromatin structure such as condensed or open chromatin states. Epigenetic modifications determine the chromatin structure partially through altering the basic subunit of DNA, the nucleosome. Accessibility of a given genomic region for active transcription can strictly depend on nucleosome positioning. Thus, mapping nucleosomes can deliver new mechanisms of regulation of gene transcription, which is discussed in Chap. 4 along with a detailed description of a methodology to determine nucleosome position and occupancy using scanning qPCR. Furthermore, nucleosome assembly is tightly associated with histone covalent modifications that have the potential to alter nucleosome positioning and occupancy. Methods for delineating histone marks and changes in histone-modifying enzymes are detailed in Chap. 5. Oncometabolites generated in cancer cells due to disrupted metabolic pathways affect the activity of histone-modifying enzymes, including Jumonji histone demethylases. This chapter elaborates on a workflow of how to assess oncometabolites' tremendous consequences for histone methylation in mammalian cells.

It becomes apparent that even active chromatin contains regions that are not transcribed. These silenced regions may be occupied by specific proteins, e.g., Polycomb group, which mediate specific histone modifications and gene silencing. On the other hand, Polycomb group-mediated gene repression can be antagonized by chromatin remodelers, e.g., BRAHMA (BRM). Hundreds of small molecule epigenetic regulators exist including derivatives of the intermediary metabolism such as adenosine triphosphate (ATP), acetyl coenzyme A (AcCoA), S-adenosyl methionine (SAM), nicotinamide adenine dinucleotide (NAD), and inositol polyphosphates (IPs). Chapter 6 presents a method for using qRT-PCR to assay the regulation of multiple genes in a 384-well format. This technology can be potentially utilized in screening for transcriptional regulators without well-defined functions that are endogenous or synthetically developed.

With Chap. 7's description of approaches for profiling expression of microRNAs, we conclude the methodology for assessing all the components of the epigenome. MicroRNAs are small noncoding RNAs that participate in post-transcriptional regulation of gene expression. Depending on their targets, microRNAs play a tumor suppressive or oncogenic role. In addition to their potential use as anticancer agents, rising evidence indicates the role of miRNAs as biomarkers for cancer. To explore their therapeutic and diagnostic potential, expression profiling in different tissues and body fluids is needed. Many miRNA profiling methods have been developed, including target-based techniques (Northern blotting, qRT-PCR, in situ hybridization [ISH]) and high-throughput methodology (microarray, RNA-Seq platforms). Chapter 7 describes target-based techniques and provides details on ISH. While Northern blotting and qRT-PCR are robust in quantifying miRNA expression in a mixture of cells from different specimens, ISH is the only imaging-based technique that takes into account expression levels along with expression heterogeneity and tissue- and cell-type specificity. Advantages and disadvantages of the methods in various applications are further discussed.

Epigenetics constitutes the interface between the environment and the genome. Numerous environmental factors have been shown to trigger changes in the epigenome including recently reported effects of gut microbiota. Gut microbial metabolites, such as butyrate or lipopolysaccharide (LPS), are known to influence the epigenome of the host and thereby regulate expression of genes involved in inflammation and fat metabolism. The workflow for compositional evaluation using qPCR and diversity analysis of microbial flora using denaturing gradient gel electrophoresis (DGGE) is detailed in Chap. 8, along with methods for studying epigenetic alterations associated with specific microbial patterns.

Most of the methods for evaluating epigenetic modifications described in Chaps. 1–8 are optimized for cell pellets, tissues, isolated nucleic acids, chromatin, etc. using an ensemble of cells. As we learn from ongoing molecular and clinical studies in the precision medicine approach, cell populations are highly heterogeneous which may impede our understanding of tested processes. There is a need for novel technology to establish connections between the molecular events in living cells, including epigenetics. Chapter 9 describes recent advances in optical microscopy and spectroscopy to capture epigenetic events in living cells. It further provides practical guidance on optical instrumentations for different applications and reviews recent advancements in sensing live-cell epigenetics. Super-resolution microscopy and Förster resonance energy transfer (FRET) are presented as methods for studying localization of target molecules and interaction. Fluorescence fluctuation spectroscopy can be applied for quantity and stoichiometry measurements whereas dynamics and kinetics can be assessed using fluorescence cross-correlation spectroscopy (FCCS), fluorescence lifetime correlation spectroscopy (FLCS), and fluorescence recovery after photobleaching (FRAP). Visualization of DNA methylation by utilizing the binding specificity between methyl-CpG-binding domain (MBD) proteins and methylated DNA is also summarized. The workflow for these techniques is complemented with advantages and disadvantages in current applications.

The book not only constitutes a resource document with advanced methodology but also delivers an extensive literature review. The last two chapters are review articles that present the current knowledge in microRNAs (miRNAs) and epigenetics of human diseases including autoimmune diseases. Chapter 10 extensively discusses the role of miRNAs in human diseases and their potential as biomarkers of drug-induced toxicity. It further demonstrates a step-by-step practical guide to identify miRNA species and test the role of miRNAs in clinically important samples using miRNA-modulating agents. In Chap. 11, readers will learn about genetics and epigenetics of multiple sclerosis, one of the most debilitating autoimmune disorders. The chapter presents an overview of how results from exome sequencing, genome-wide association studies, transcriptome, and epigenome mapping contribute to deciphering the pathophysiology, progression, and different subtypes of the disease.

Finally, we are grateful to all the contributors for their tremendous efforts to prepare the chapters and to share their knowledge in various aspects of epigenetics and gene expression studies in cancer, inflammatory and immune diseases. It was a great pleasure and invaluable experience to work with each of them.

West Lafayette, IA, USA   *Barbara Stefanska*
Liverpool, UK   *David J. MacEwan*

Contents

Contributors

DANIEL J. ANTOINE • *Department of Molecular and Clinical Pharmacology, Institute of Translational Medicine, University of Liverpool, Liverpool, UK*

HUNTER T. BALDUF • *Department of Biochemistry, and Purdue Center for Cancer Research, Purdue University, West Lafayette, IN, USA*

RUCHI BANSAL • *Department of Medical and Molecular Genetics, Indiana University School of Medicine (IUSM), Indianapolis, IN, USA*

LEIGH C. CARMODY • *Center for the Development of Therapeutics, Broad Institute of Harvard and MIT, Cambridge, MA, USA*

DAVID CHEISHVILI • *Department of Pharmacology and Therapeutics, McGill University Medical School, Montreal, QC, Canada*

STEFFAN CHRISTIANSEN • *Department of Biomedicine, Aarhus University, Aarhus, Denmark*

YI CUI • *Department of Agricultural and Biological Engineering, Bindley Bioscience Centre, Purdue Center for Cancer Research, Purdue University, West Lafayette, IN, USA*

PRASAD P. DEVARSHI • *Department of Nutrition Science, Purdue University, West Lafayette, IN, USA*

EMILY C. DYKHUIZEN • *Department of Medicinal Chemistry and Molecular Pharmacology, Purdue University, West Lafayette, IN, USA*

MARTINA GREUNZ • *Department of Nutritional Sciences, University Vienna, Vienna, Austria*

ALEXANDER G. HASLBERGER • *Department of Nutritional Sciences, University Vienna, Vienna, Austria*

TARA M. HENAGAN • *Department of Nutrition Science, Purdue University, West Lafayette, IN, USA*

ATIF HUSSAIN • *Department of Biological Sciences, Centre for Environmental Epigenetics and Development, University of Toronto Scarborough, Toronto, ON, Canada*

JOSEPH IRUDAYARAJ • *Department of Agricultural and Biological Engineering, Bindley Bioscience Centre, Purdue Center for Cancer Research, Purdue University, West Lafayette, IN, USA*

HEIDRUN KARLIC • *Ludwig Boltzmann Institute for Leukemia Research and Hematology, Hanusch Hospital, Vienna, Austria*

ANN L. KIRCHMAIER • *Department of Biochemistry, Purdue University, West Lafayette, IN, USA; Purdue Center for Cancer Research, Purdue University, West Lafayette, IN, USA*

MURRAY KORC • *Department of Biochemistry and Molecular Biology, IUSM, Indianapolis, IN, USA; The Melvin and Bren Simon Cancer Center, IUSM, Indianapolis, IN, USA; Pancreatic Cancer Signature Center, Indiana University and Purdue University-Indianapolis (IUPUI), Indianapolis, IN, USA*

JANAIAH KOTA • *Department of Medical and Molecular Genetics, Indiana University School of Medicine (IUSM), Indianapolis, IN, USA; The Melvin and Bren Simon Cancer Center, IUSM, Indianapolis, IN, USA; Pancreatic Cancer Signature Center, Indiana University and Purdue University-Indianapolis (IUPUI), Indianapolis, IN, USA*

JASON KWON • *Department of Medical and Molecular Genetics, Indiana University School of Medicine (IUSM), Indianapolis, IN, USA*

LUCA LOVREČIČ • *Department of Obstetrics and Gynecology, Clinical Institute of Medical Genetics, University Medical Center Ljubljana, Ljubljana, Slovenia*

VIDMAR LOVRO • *Department of Obstetrics and Gynecology, Clinical Institute of Medical Genetics, University Medical Center Ljubljana, Ljubljana, Slovenia*

DAVID J. MACEWAN • *Department of Molecular and Clinical Pharmacology, Institute of Translational Medicine, University of Liverpool, Liverpool, UK*

ALES MAVER • *Department of Obstetrics and Gynecology, Clinical Institute of Medical Genetics, University Medical Center Ljubljana, Ljubljana, Slovenia*

PATRICK O. MCGOWAN • *Department of Biological Sciences, Centre for Environmental Epigenetics and Development, University of Toronto Scarborough, Toronto, ON, Canada; Department of Cell and Systems Biology, University of Toronto, Toronto, ON, Canada; Department of Psychology, University of Toronto, Toronto, ON, Canada; Department of Physiology, University of Toronto, Toronto, ON, Canada*

ANTONELLA PEPE • *Purdue Center for Cancer Research, Purdue University, West Lafayette, IN, USA*

BORUT PETERLIN • *Department of Obstetrics and Gynecology, Clinical Institute of Medical Genetics, University Medical Center Ljubljana, Ljubljana, Slovenia*

SOPHIE PETROPOULOS • *Department of Clinical Science, Intervention and Technology (CLINTEC), Karolinska Institutet, Stockholm, Sweden*

IRENE REBHAN • *Department of Nutritional Sciences, University Vienna, Vienna, Austria*

MARLENE REMELY • *Department of Nutritional Sciences, University Vienna, Vienna, Austria*

NIRAJ M. SHAH • *Department of Molecular and Clinical Pharmacology, Institute of Translational Medicine, University of Liverpool, Liverpool, UK*

MOSHE SZYF • *Department of Pharmacology and Therapeutics, McGill University Medical School, Montreal, QC, Canada*

ANUSHA THOTA • *Department of Medical and Molecular Genetics, Indiana University School of Medicine (IUSM), Indianapolis, IN, USA*

NICOLA J. TOLLIDAY • *Center for the Development of Therapeutics, Broad Institute of Harvard and MIT, Cambridge, MA, USA*

WILFRED C. DE VEGA • *Department of Biological Sciences, Centre for Environmental Epigenetics and Development, University of Toronto Scarborough, Toronto, ON, Canada; Department of Cell and Systems Biology, University of Toronto, Toronto, ON, Canada*

SUSHUMA YARLAGADDA • *Department of Medical and Molecular Genetics, Indiana University School of Medicine (IUSM), Indianapolis, IN, USA*

Chapter 1

High-Throughput Techniques for DNA Methylation Profiling

Sophie Petropoulos, David Cheishvili, and Moshe Szyf

Abstract

In this chapter, commonly used methods to assess the genome wide DNA methylation status are reviewed and compared. The methods described in this chapter include enrichment-based method, Methylated DNA Immunoprecipitation (MeDIP), paired with microarray technology and next generation sequencing, and sodium bisulfate-based techniques including Infinium HumanMethylation450 BeadChip (Illumina 450 K) and Reduced Representation Bisulfite Sequencing (RRBS).

An overview of each protocol, including description as to why particular steps are required or critical, is outlined. Further, the protocols are compared and advantages and disadvantages of each are discussed.

Key words DNA methylation, Sodium bisulfite, Methylated DNA immunoprecipitation (MeDIP), Infinium HumanMethylation450 BeadChip (Illumina 450 K), Reduced Representation Bisulfite Sequencing (RRBS), Microarray, Next generation sequencing

1   Introduction

The haploid human genome contains approximately 28 million CpG sites [1], which may potentially be differentially methylated. DNA methylation is an enzymatic covalent modification of DNA that does not alter the nucleotide sequence itself. Methyltransferases (DNMT1, DNTM3a, and DNMT3b) catalyze and maintain the transfer of a methyl moiety to the 5′ position of the cytosine ring [2–5]. DNA methylation plays an essential and dynamic role in regulating gene expression, which can include directly blocking the binding of transcription factors to elements containing a methylated CpG dinucleotide [6], or indirectly through recruitment of methylated DNA binding factors [7], which in turn recruit histone deacetylases and methyltransferases to inactivate the chromatin [8, 9].

In the mammalian genome, DNA methylation is primarily present in CpG dinucleotides dispersed throughout the genome (non-CpG islands), but may also occur at non-CpG sites (CpHpG, H = A, T, C). Location of the methylated cytosine is critical for

Barbara Stefanska and David J. MacEwan (eds.), *Epigenetics and Gene Expression in Cancer, Inflammatory and Immune Diseases*, Methods In Pharmacology and Toxicology, DOI 10.1007/978-1-4939-6743-8_1, © Springer Science+Business Media LLC 2017

gene expression. While DNA methylation in the promoter inversely correlates with gene expression, the role of DNA methylation in the gene body and intragenic regions is still under investigation. Some recent papers report a direct correlation between DNA methylation in the gene body and associated gene expression [10–12].

Accurate assessment of DNA methylation is critical for obtaining accurate data and for better understanding of disease, cellular processes, development, and pluripotency. Emerging evidence supports the hypothesis that modulation to the methylome plays a key role in a broad spectrum of chronic diseases. DNA methylation has been shown to regulate autoimmunity and immunity. For example, dendritic cell differentiation and activation as well as monocyte/macrophage differentiation have been shown to be regulated by DNA methylation [13, 14]. DNA methylation is implicated in autoimmune diseases such as systemic lupus erythematosus, rheumatoid arthritis, multiple sclerosis, and type 1 diabetes mellitus [15]. Moreover, though a genetic basis has been demonstrated to contribute to the etiology of disease, gene-environment interactions mediated by the methylome may also explain the onset and/or development of diseases such as neurodegeneration and various cancers [16–20]. The increasing evidence supporting a role of DNA methylation in the molecular pathology of chronic disease highlights the need for robust technologies to accurately detect and quantify changes to the methylome.

To date, multiple high-throughput techniques are available for assessing DNA methylation and determining differentially methylated regions (DMRs), making it difficult to decide which technology to use. DNA methylation analyses methods can be generally classified into region-based and site-based resolution. The example of region-based DNA methylation includes: Methylated DNA Immunoprecipitation (MeDIP)-seq and MeDIP-ChIP, while whole-genome bisulfite sequencing, Reduced Representation Bisulfite Sequencing (RRBS), and Illumina Infinium HumanMethylation450 BeadChip (Illumina 450 K) are examples of base-specific resolution assays. Each technique has innate biases, pros, and cons and one must determine which would best suit their study. In this chapter, we will highlight the three most commonly used genome-wide techniques and elaborate on the pros and cons associated with each method: MeDIP-seq and RRBS, high-throughput next generation sequencing, these techniques that provide high throughput, partly comprehensive genome-wide data pertaining to the methylome. MeDIP-ChIP and Illumina BeadChip 450 K are microarray-based approaches and in general provide lower coverage [21].

2 Methylated DNA Immunoprecipitation (MeDIP)

MeDIP is a method that captures the relative enrichment of methylated DNA across a genome by utilizing an antibody that binds to 5-methyl-cytosine (5mc)[22–24]. This platform was utilized to delineate the first genome-wide mammalian methylome.

High quality, RNA and protein-free genomic DNA is crucial for optimal results. The specificity and efficiency of antibody binding and thus immunoprecipitation may be affected by contaminated and degraded genomic DNA. As such, numerous precautions should be taken to assess quality prior to commencing with the immunoprecipitation. Both commercial kits and the standard phenol–chloroform extraction work well to obtain high quality genomic DNA. Following isolation, quantity and quality should be measured. Typically, Nanodrop or a spectrophotometer is used to measure the 260/280 UV absorbance ratio, which provides a measure of DNA purity. A ratio of ~1.8 is considered to be ideal. It is also recommended to check for additional contaminants such as EDTA and phenol by measuring the 260/230 UV absorbance ratio; pure nucleic acid should give a ratio of 2.0–2.2. Finally, it is also recommended to run samples on agarose gel electrophoresis stained with ethidium bromide to ensure clean, high molecular weight bands as opposed to smears, which would indicate degradation. A minimum of 2 µg of starting genomic DNA is recommended to proceed with either MeDIP-seq or MeDIP-ChIP. For a protocol overview, please see schematic in Fig. 1a.

Following quantification and quality control, genomic DNA must be randomly fragmented between 250 and 1000 bp [24]. Bioruptor® (Diagenode) is recommended with 8 cycles of 5 s on/15 s off; however, the duration and number of cycles may need to be adjusted. Gel electrophoresis should be performed following sonication to confirm size of fragments of sheared DNA. Following genomic DNA shearing, the sample is boiled and immediately placed on ice to denature into single-strands. From this portion, an aliquot is removed and frozen for later use which represents the "input." Following this, the remaining sample is precleared and incubated with 5mC antibody and incubated overnight. Postincubation, the sample is washed and resuspended; this represents the "bound" fraction.

To assess the efficacy of the immunoprecipitation prior to proceeding with downstream applications. qPCR, comparing the bound fraction to input for specific loci, is often performed. The promoter of imprinted genes, such as *H19*, is commonly used as a "positive" control normalized to housekeeping genes, such as *GAPDH*, which have minimal or no methylation. Alternatively, spiking samples with unmethylated plasmid and a methylated different plasmid (6 pg of each) prior to sonication is advisable.

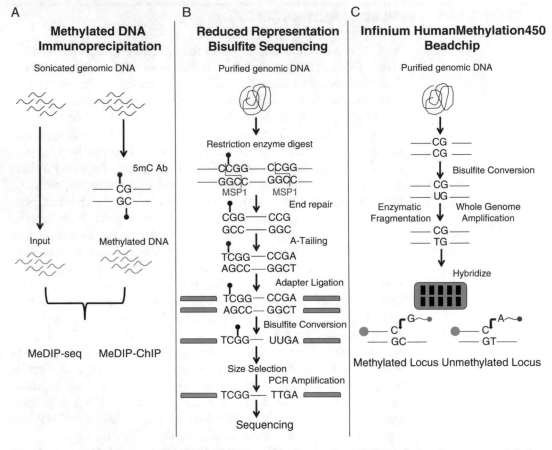

Fig. 1 Schematic of high-throughput methodologies outlined in chapter. (**a**) DNA Methylated Immunoprecipitation, (**b**) Reduced Representation Bisulfite Sequencing, and (**c**) Infinium HumanMethylation450 BeadChip

Following immunoprecipitation, qPCR with specific primers can be performed on unmethylated and methylated plasmids to validate enrichment for methylated DNA in bound fractions. Additional spike-in approaches are available [25]. Enrichment (E) can be calculated as follows; $E = (B_{target}/I_{target})/(B_{negative\ control}/I_{negative\ control})$ where "target" is the methylated region of interest and "negative control" is an unmethylated DNA region.

Numerous downstream applications of MeDIP are currently available, both for interrogating DNA methylation at a single loci (see Chap. 3) and genome-wide. Initially, MeDIP was paired with microarray technology (MeDIP-ChIP) [24]; however, this requires micrograms of DNA, which is not always feasible depending on the biological sample. With next generation sequencing, as little as 1–50 ng of DNA can be sufficient [26, 27]. Further, next generation sequencing has allowed for a more efficient and cheaper platform compared to hybridization to microarrays.

The protocol described needs to be modified slightly depending on the specific downstream application chosen. For example, for MeDIP-seq, sonicated DNA needs to be end-repaired, A-tailed and ligated with Illumina adapters [28, 29]. Samples are then gel-excised to enrich for only adapter-ligated DNA prior to proceeding with immunoprecipitation [25, 26]. In contrast, for MeDIP-ChIP, input and bound fractions can be whole-genome amplified (WGA) and then labeled with Cy3 and Cy5 dye for co-hybridization on microarray platforms [24, 26].

A general drawback of using MeDIP approach to assess DNA methylation, as with any enrichment-based methodologies, is resolution. Given that DNA is sheared into fragments, it is impossible to differentiate if one or more of the CpGs present is responsible for the antibody binding and whether non-CpG methylation is present; thus, this method has relatively low resolution. In addition, enriched fragments are biased by variables such as CpG density, making it difficult to ascertain absolute methylation [30]. However, given that the methylation status of CpGs within 1000 bp sequence is significantly correlated, a lower resolution (~100–150 bp) as with MeDIP-seq/MeDIP-ChIP could be suitable despite absence of single-CpG information [23]. Nonetheless, to circumvent the resolution issue, a computational model (methylCRF algorithm) has been recently developed to extrapolate data derived from MeDIP-seq to predict methylation at single-CpG resolution [31].

2.1 MeDIP-ChIP

Initially, MeDIP was paired with microarrays and is often referred to as MeDIP-ChIP. A variety of microarray designs are available that range in coverage both by depth and region and number of samples that can be hybridized (microarrays per slide). The most popular companies supplying microarrays are Agilent, NimbleGen, and Affymetrix, and each offers minor differences in their array designs. In general, Targeted, Custom, and Tiled arrays are commonly used designs for the study of DNA methylation. Targeted arrays allocate the probes within specific regions of the genome such as CpG islands (covering ~27 000 CpG islands, CGIs) or gene promoters. For promoter arrays, the probe placement is a few Kb both upstream and downstream from the transcription start site (TSS) of known RefSeq transcripts. Tiled arrays, on the other hand, distribute the probes throughout the genome and are not limited to known target sequences, and thus contain less bias than traditional Target arrays. Further, coverage with tiling arrays can be adjusted depending on probe placement. For example, probes can be spaced with no overlap, overlap of a few base pairs, or almost complete overlap, which offers the highest resolution. Custom arrays can also be designed which can for example enrich for a specific gene list, or combine a promoter and tiled array design.

This design is beneficial if a list of preexisting target genes are of interest in addition to the identification of potentially novel regions/genes that may be differentially methylated.

Another aspect of array design to consider is the tradeoff between the number of probes (which translates to genome coverage) versus the number of arrays per slide, where generally one array corresponds to one biological sample. For example, Agilent offers SurePrint G3 arrays ranging from 1X 1 M, which is comprised of one array/slide and one million probes, to 8× 60 K which is comprised of eight arrays/slide and 60,000 probes. Depending on one's budget, sample size, and coverage needs, researchers have the flexibility to choose a slide design that best suits their needs.

Drawbacks associated with using microarray platform for MeDIP are nonspecific hybrization and background noise [32, 33], which require intensive normalization. Further, regardless of array design, coverage of the genome is still limited since oligonucleotide probes must be pre-designed and are reliant on known genomic sequences. Finally, the low amount of immunoprecipitated fraction requires whole genome amplification (WGA) prior to hybridization, which may introduce bias for CpG-rich promoters [34]. Nonetheless, very pertinent data regarding DNA methylation can be generated at relatively low costs using array hybridization, making this platform cost-efficient and reproducible.

2.2 MeDIP-Seq

With the emergence of next generation sequencing, MeDIP-seq was developed [29]. Though both MeDIP-Chip and MeDIP-seq are enrichment-based approaches, unlike microarray platforms where coverage is based on a-priory probe design, MeDIP-seq provided a greater coverage genome-wide, with >97% of methylated regions being detected [29]. In comparison to other methods, MeDIP-seq's coverage genome-wide is superior (~20×), with a detection of ~60% of all CpG sites in the human genome, and ~90% of all CpG sites present in regulatory regions and CGIs [29].

Overall, MeDIP-seq does appear to be the most cost efficient for genome-wide CpG coverage [28, 35].

3 Reduced Representation Bisulfite Sequencing

Reduced Representation Bisulfite Sequencing (RRBS) methodology was developed in 2005, originally as a random shotgun bisulfite sequencing approach [36]. It utilized restriction enzymes to fragment the genomic DNA and enrich for CpG containing motifs, which is then size selected and thus generates a "reduced representation" of the genome [36]. Since CpG methylation status is measured in regions that are only CpG dense, approximately 3 Gb of sequencing is required to obtain approximately equal sequencing depth among regions of interest [21, 28].

Unlike MeDIP that is an enrichment-based technique relying on antibody binding, RRBS is based on bisulfite sequencing, currently considered the gold standard for assessing DNA methylation [37]. Bisulfite sequencing is based on the principle that an unmethylated cytosine is deaminated following bisulfite treatment and converted into uracil. The DNA is single stranded and DNA polymerase then generates the complimentary strand, in which a methylated cytosine reads as cytosine and the unmethylated cytosine reads as thymine. Today, RRBS is a high-throughput genome-wide platform to efficiently assess DNA methylation.

Sodium bisulfite treatment is harsh and is believed to cause >90% degradation of DNA [38] and potentially introduce mutations to the DNA sequence [27], thus affecting the DNA sequence and reliability of the readout. Another inherent drawback of bisulfite sequencing is the possibility of incomplete conversion due to incomplete DNA denaturation or re-annealing and thus being able to decipher whether a "methylated" cytosine is truly methylated or a technical artifact. Further, misrepresentation of specific sequences can occur due to PCR amplification bias [36]. Nonetheless, results from RRBS are highly reproducible and cytosine conversion rates are >99.9% [36, 39].

A major benefit of RRBS is the low starting input of DNA required, allowing for this approach to be applied to single-cell analysis of the methylome, single-cell Reduced Representation Bisulfite Sequencing (sc-RRBS) [39]. In this protocol, the purification steps required have been reduced to one, minimizing the loss of DNA. All the steps preceding sequencing are performed in a single tube. The coverage of sc-RRBS compared to RRBS is lower, but nonetheless impressive at ~40% overlap of CpG sites captured by RRBS. Given the heterogeneity in cell populations, further development of single-cell techniques exploring the epigenome would provide a wealth of data and push forward the knowledge in numerous fields of study.

The general workflow for RRBS includes extraction of high quality genomic DNA, similar to what was described above. DNA methylation regions are then targeted by Msp1 digestion, which captures a representation of the genome. The digested DNA then undergoes gap filling and A-tailing and is digested and size selected by gel-based exclusion or SPRI bead purification (40–220 bp). Illumina adapters are then ligated to allow pooling of samples. The pooled DNA is then bisulfite converted, size selected, and sequenced with next generation sequencing platform. Detailed comprehensive protocols for RRBS are widely available [36, 40–42]. Please see Fig. 1b for a schematic of protocol.

Recently, a novel, user-friendly web service was developed to assist with the analysis and alignment of bisulfite sequencing data, Web Service for Bisulfite Sequencing Data Analysis (WBSA), http://wbsa.big.ac.cn [43]. WBSA is comparable to pre-existing bioinformatics tools and in addition incorporates non-CpG methylation alignment, and therefore is appealing to a broader scientific community [43]. Minimizing the complexities associated with data analysis, web services such as WBSA is only one example of how high-throughput techniques can be more easily incorporated into laboratories' workflow.

4   Infinium HumanMethylation450 BeadChip Array

Along with RRBS, Infinium HumanMethylation450 BeadChip array (Illumina 450 K) (Illumina, Inc. CA, USA) enables the researcher to assess single base-pair DNA methylation. Illumina 450 K is a relatively new method, which has replaced the previous generation 27 K Infinium methylation array. Compared to Illumina 27 K, which targeted mostly promoter sites and covered only 27578 CpGs associated with 14495 genes, Illumina 450 K methylation array is used to quantify the methylation status of over 480,000 cytosines in human genome. It covers around 99 % of RefSeq genes, with an average of 17 CpG sites per gene. While the role of DNA methylation in promoter and CpG island is widely accepted, the importance of DNA methylation in gene body or shore regions for transcription regulation has recently come to attention [44, 45]. Illumina, Inc., (San Diego, CA, USA) in the guidance of a consortium of methylation experts comprising 22 members that represent 19 institutions worldwide develop the Infinium HumanMethylation450 BeadChip, which in addition to the promoter regions (including multiple sites in the annotated promoter regions, 1500 and 200 bp upstream of transcription start site) includes CpG sites localized in 5'UTR, first exon, gene body, and 3'UTR. Illumina 450 K covers 96 % of CpG islands, with additional coverage in island shores and the regions flanking them. In addition, Illumina 450 K microarray includes non-CpG sites outside of CpGs islands and miRNA promoter regions. The significantly increased coverage, high reproducibility across other platforms ($r = 0.88$ with Pyrosequencing) [1, 46], along with relatively low cost, make Illumina 450 K an attractive and powerful platform in epigenome-wide association studies (EWAS).

4.1 Technical Requirement

Genomic DNA samples for Illumina 450 K can be extracted using classical phenol-chloroform method or any other DNA extraction procedure. DNA should be diluted either in 1X TE buffer (10 mM Tris–HCl pH 8.0/1 mM EDTA) or in nuclease-free water. It is preferable to measure DNA concentration by PicoGreen DNA Measurement and adjusted to the range of about 70–130 ng/μl. Typically, 500 ng input of genomic DNA is sufficient [47]. It is highly recommended to assess DNA sample integrity by agarose gel electrophoresis to ensure that there is no degradation.

The purity of each DNA sample from proteins or other organic compounds should be verified using A260/A280 and A260/A230 ratios, using UV-Vis spectrophotometer or NanoDrop. A260/A280 absorbance ratio should be from 1.8 to 2.0, and A260/A230 ratio should be >2.0. It is also recommended to randomize DNA samples on a 96-well plate to minimize position biases [48].

4.2   Illumina 450 K Array Overview

Each Illumina 450 K BeadChip array has a 12 DNA sample format. In total, 96 DNA samples can be run in parallel. The whole process takes about 3 days, and includes the following steps: first, about 500 ng of DNA is subjected to bisulfite conversion (which converts all unmethylated cytosines into uracil, while methylated cytosines remain unchanged), followed by additional quality control to ensure the efficiency of bisulfite conversion. After DNA bisulfite conversion, the analysis of DNA methylation is reduced to an analysis of single nucleotide polymorphisms (SNPs). For a schematic of the protocol, see Fig. 1c.

Illumina Infinium HumanMethylation450 BeadChip (450 K) is based on the Infinium Technology. Compared to the older 27 K methylation array, which used only Infinium type 1 probes, Illumina 450 K utilizes two different types of chemical assays (Infinium I and Infinium II), which are dispensed randomly across the array [49], and are based on analysis of single nucleotide polymorphism (SNP) for T's and C's generated by bisulfite conversion. The Infinium I assay (one third of array cytosines) uses two different probes, located on two different bead types. One is for the methylated locus (M bead type) and another is for the unmethylated locus (U bead type). Compared to Infinium I, Infinium II assay design (two thirds of array cytosines) requires only one probe per locus, allowing detection of both alleles, methylated and non-methylated. Using two different assays (Infinium I and Infinium II) allows coverage of many more cytosine compared to Illumina 27 K; however, this causes a difference in distribution of β-values (see below), derived from these two designs. Infinium II β-values were reported to be less accurate for the detection of extreme methylation values, than those obtained from Infinium I probes [49, 50], which is probably associated with the dual-channel readout, thus rendering the Infinium I assay a better estimator of the true methylation state.

To assess and analyze the biological variability in DNA methylation, it is essential to minimize technical variability, batch effects, and bias. To correct this, few R statistical computing software associated packages were developed. Peak-based correction (PBC) [49] normalizes type 2 design probes to make them comparable with type 1 probes. Subset-quantile Within Array Normalization (SWAN) allows the Infinium I and II probes within a single array to be normalized together. SWAN substantially reduces the differences in β value distribution observed between Infinium I and II probes, improves correlation between technical replicates, while increasing the number of significantly differentially methylated probes that are detected (SWAN is available in the minfi R package) [51, 52]. Recently, novel normalization strategy Beta MIxture Quantile dilation (BMIQ) [53] has been proposed, which is set as a default method of normalization in ChAMP package [54]. Other normalization methods include quantile normalization [50, 51], dasen [55], and noob [56].

4.3 Illumina 450 K Data Analysis

Two methods have been proposed to measure methylation level, beta-value, and M-value [57]. Beta value, which is a more popular way of DNA methylation representation, estimates the methylation level using intensity ratio between methylated and unmethylated alleles. It ranges from 0 to 1 and measures actually the percentage of methylation (when $\beta = 0$, all cells are non-methylated, and when $\beta = 1$, all cells are methylated). M-value is a log2 ratio of methylated and unmethylated probes intensity. Though Illumina recommends by default, using Beta-value to assess DNA methylation level [58, 59], some reports show that M-value is more statistically valid, while beta value has severe heteroscedasticity for highly methylated or unmethylated CpG sites.

There are free R associated software available to convert Beta to M value, Lumi [57], and Methylumi [60]. The sample size is one of the parameters that can affect value selection. It was reported that when the sample size is relatively large, feature selection using test statistics is similar for M and β-values, but that in small sample size studies, M-values allow more reliable identification of true positives [61]. Multiple methods have been proposed for analysis of data generated by Illumina 450 K methylation bead-chip array [49, 50, 54, 62–64]. Along with site-specific-based methods, alternative region-based methods can also be applied. The Probe Lasso, which is implemented in the R package ChAMP [54], represents a DMR (differential methylated region) calling method that gathers neighboring significant signals to define clear DMRs [65].

Along with obvious advantages, Illumina 450 K bead array was reported to carry some major disadvantages including the following: only human samples can currently be analyzed, it cannot distinguish between 5-hydroxymethylcytosine from 5-methylcytosine and custom probe design is not an option. Further, in a recent study, it was reported that 6% of the Illumina 450 K microarray probes are cross-reactive, co-hybridizing to alternate sequences highly homologous to the intended targets, non-targeted genomic regions, or target loci that contain known SNPs. They report that 49.3% of all sites have a probe that overlaps with at least one SNP [66]. All these should be taken into account when analyzing Illumina 450 K data and also considering use of this platform.

5   Comparison of Methods

5-methylcytosine in the context of CpG dinucleotide is one of the most studied epigenetic marks, with an increased interest in investigating its biological function over the last three decades. As such, choosing the "best" platform to investigate this chemical modification for your specific study is of importance for the generation of robust and accurate data.

MeDIP-seq and MeDIP-ChIP rely on the use of an antibody to enrich the DNA methylated fraction, while RRBS and Illumina450K use bisulfite conversion of genomic DNA. For enrichment-based approach, data is not biased by a specific nucleotide sequence as occurs with restriction enzyme methods (e.g., RRBS); however, RRBS and Illumina 450 K have been shown to not require statistical correction for CpG bias and overall tend to provide a more accurate measure to detect DMRs [21]. In contrast, regions with minimal or no methylation and CpG poor regions are generally excluded from MeDIP-seq, thus providing low statistical power compared to RRBS and Infinium [21]. In contrast, Illumina 450 K may be effective at assessing CpG-poor regions (CpGs island shores and shelves), which have been shown to be particularly susceptible to altered DNA-methylation in response to environmental exposure and carcinogenesis [44].

These methods also differ with regard to resolution. MeDIP has relatively low resolution given that DNA is sheared into fragments, and based on the enrichment of fragments, making it difficult to measure absolute methylation [30]. However, another aspect to consider is that the higher resolution obtained with RRBS and Infinum has a tradeoff with lower coverage of the genome compared to MeDIP-seq [21]. Further, though MeDIP-seq and Illumina 450 K have shown overall good correlation with regard to detection of overlapping CpG sites, regions with poor correlation do exist and are likely a result of the poorer resolution in enrichment-based protocols [35]. Illumina 450 K has few advantages over other genome-wide methods, such as relatively low cost per sample and broad coverage of representative CpGs across the human genome. Though Illumina 450 K bead chip array only assays approximately 1.8 % of CpGs, which is much less than other genome-wide methods, it is highly amenable to studying large sample sizes, which may be critical when considering statistical power.

With regard to coverage, discrepancies do exist among these techniques. For example, given that approximately 45 % of the human genome contains repetitive elements with a large proportion of CpGs, MeDIP-seq is advantageous over MeDIP-ChIP, which cannot interrogate CpGs located in transposable elements [23, 28]. In a comparative study, MeDIP-seq and RRBS were found comparable in their detections of DMRs in repetitive sequences using two complementary approaches for analysis [21]. Further, in a comparison examining the percent coverage of repetitive elements with Illumina 450 K methylation and MeDIP-seq, MeDIP-seq provided 94 % more coverage [35]. However, MeDIP-seq had the lowest detection level of genome-wide DMRs when compared to RRBS and Infinium [21]. Further, CpG islands are relatively unmethylated so enrichment-based methods tend to provide lower coverage of CGIs when compared to other methods such as RRBS [28]. A comparison of MeDIP-seq, RRBS, and Infinium showed that MeDIP-seq was not as robust in determining DNA methylation of partially methylated regions [28]. In contrast, Illumina 450 K tends to underestimate methylation level in semi or highly methylated regions [35].

6   Conclusion

With the advancement of new technologies, genome-wide DNA methylation mapping has become accessible to a broader range of laboratories. Interrogating the methylome in disease, development, and pluripotency is of interest for the development of therapeutics, establishing biomarkers and obtaining a comprehensive understanding of the underlying biological processes. The methodologies highlighted in this chapter are among the most commonly used today. Overall, the methods outlined do overlap with detection ability of DMRs; however, discrepancies exist when examining CpG poor regions, CGIs and repeat elements. RRBS and Illumina 450 K are both bisulfate-based methods that measure absolute methylation, whereas MeDIP-seq and MeDIP-ChIP are enrichment-based methods and thus only provide information on the relative abundance of DNA methylation. Deciding on which particular approach to utilize is often difficult and one must consider all the biases, cost, sample size, and confounding factors associated with each technique and how it best suits their particular study. Another consideration is the allocation of resources between sequencing depth or increased biological sample sequencing. Overall, these techniques have proven to be accurate in determining DNA methylation levels despite the minor discrepancies.

Acknowledgments

S.P. is supported by the Mats Sundin Fellowship in Developmental Health. D. C. is supported by fellowship from the Israel Cancer Research Foundation.

References

1. Bibikova M, Barnes B, Tsan C et al (2011) High density DNA methylation array with single CpG site resolution. Genomics 98:288–295

2. Gold M, Gefter M, Hausmann R, Hurwitz J (1966) Methylation of DNA. J Gen Physiol 49:5–28

3. Razin A, Riggs AD (1980) DNA methylation and gene function. Science 210:604–610

4. Li E, Bestor TH, Jaenisch R (1992) Targeted mutation of the DNA methyltransferase gene results in embryonic lethality. Cell 69:915–926

5. Okano M, Bell DW, Haber DA, Li E (1999) DNA methyltransferases Dnmt3a and Dnmt3b are essential for de novo methylation and mammalian development. Cell 99:247–257

6. Comb M, Goodman HM (1990) CpG methylation inhibits proenkephalin gene expression and binding of the transcription factor AP-2. Nucleic Acids Res 18:3975–3982

7. Lewis JD, Meehan RR, Henzel WJ et al (1992) Purification, sequence, and cellular localization of a novel chromosomal protein that binds to methylated DNA. Cell 69:905–914

8. Jones PL, Veenstra GJ, Wade PA et al (1998) Methylated DNA and MeCP2 recruit histone deacetylase to repress transcription. Nat Genet 19:187–191

9. Nan X, Ng HH, Johnson CA et al (1998) Transcriptional repression by the methyl-CpG-binding protein MeCP2 involves a histone deacetylase complex. Nature 393:386–389

10. Yang X, Han H, De Carvalho DD, Lay FD, Jones PA, Liang G (2014) Gene body methylation can alter gene expression and is a therapeutic target in cancer. Cancer Cell 26:577–590

11. Jjingo D, Conley AB, Yi SV, Lunyak VV, Jordan IK (2012) On the presence and role of human gene-body DNA methylation. Oncotarget 3:462–474

12. Schultz MD, He Y, Whitaker JW et al (2015) Human body epigenome maps reveal noncanonical DNA methylation variation. Nature 523:212–216

13. Zhao M, Liu S, Luo S et al (2014) DNA methylation and mRNA and microRNA expression of SLE CD4+ T cells correlate with disease phenotype. J Autoimmun 54:127–136

14. Karpurapu M, Ranjan R, Deng J et al (2014) Krüppel like factor 4 promoter undergoes active demethylation during monocyte/macrophage differentiation. PLoS One 9, e93362

15. Zhao M, Wang Z, Yung S, Lu Q (2015) Epigenetic dynamics in immunity and autoimmunity. Int J Biochem Cell Biol 67:65–74

16. Lardenoije R, Iatrou A, Kenis G et al (2015) The epigenetics of aging and neurodegeneration. Prog Neurobiol 131:21–64

17. Landgrave-Gómez J, Mercado-Gómez O, Guevara-Guzmán R (2015) Epigenetic mechanisms in neurological and neurodegenerative diseases. Front Cell Neurosci 9:58

18. Paska AV, Hudler P (2015) Aberrant methylation patterns in cancer: a clinical view. Biochem Medica 25:161–176

19. Chiang N-J, Shan Y-S, Hung W-C, Chen L-T (2015) Epigenetic regulation in the carcinogenesis of cholangiocarcinoma. Int J Biochem Cell Biol 67:110–114

20. Sui X, Zhu J, Zhou J et al (2015) Epigenetic modifications as regulatory elements of autophagy in cancer. Cancer Lett 360:106–113

21. Bock C, Tomazou EM, Brinkman AB et al (2010) Quantitative comparison of genome-wide DNA methylation mapping technologies. Nat Biotechnol 28:1106–1114

22. Laird PW (2010) Principles and challenges of genomewide DNA methylation analysis. Nat Rev Genet 11:191–203

23. Beck S, Rakyan VK (2008) The methylome: approaches for global DNA methylation profiling. Trends Genet 24:231–237

24. Weber M, Davies JJ, Wittig D et al (2005) Chromosome-wide and promoter-specific analyses identify sites of differential DNA methylation in normal and transformed human cells. Nat Genet 37:853–862

25. Lisanti S, von Zglinicki T, Mathers JC (2012) Standardization and quality controls for the methylated DNA immunoprecipitation technique. Epigenetics 7:615–625

26. Borgel J, Guibert S, Weber M (2012) Methylated DNA immunoprecipitation (MeDIP) from low amounts of cells. Methods Mol Biol 925:149–158

27. Zhao M-T, Whyte JJ, Hopkins GM, Kirk MD, Prather RS (2014) Methylated DNA immunoprecipitation and high-throughput sequencing (MeDIP-seq) using low amounts of genomic DNA. Cell Reprogram 16:175–184

28. Harris RA, Wang T, Coarfa C et al (2010) Comparison of sequencing-based methods to profile DNA methylation and identification of monoallelic epigenetic modifications. Nat Biotechnol 28:1097–1105

29. Down TA, Rakyan VK, Turner DJ et al (2008) A Bayesian deconvolution strategy for immunoprecipitation-based DNA methylome analysis. Nat Biotechnol 26:779–785

30. Pelizzola M, Koga Y, Urban AE et al (2008) MEDME: an experimental and analytical methodology for the estimation of DNA methylation levels based on microarray derived MeDIP-enrichment. Genome Res 18:1652–1659

31. Stevens M, Cheng JB, Li D et al (2013) Estimating absolute methylation levels at single-CpG resolution from methylation enrichment and restriction enzyme sequencing methods. Genome Res 23:1541–1553

32. Otto C, Reiche K, Hackermuller J (2012) Detection of differentially expressed segments in tiling array data. Bioinformatics 28:1471–1479

33. Sorek R, Cossart P (2010) Prokaryotic transcriptomics: a new view on regulation, physiology and pathogenicity. Nat Rev Genet 11: 9–16

34. Jia J, Pekowska A, Jaeger S, Benoukraf T, Ferrier P, Spicuglia S (2010) Assessing the efficiency and significance of Methylated DNA Immunoprecipitation (MeDIP) assays in using in vitro methylated genomic DNA. BMC Res Notes 3:240

35. Clark C, Palta P, Joyce CJ et al (2012) A comparison of the whole genome approach of MeDIP-seq to the targeted approach of the Infinium HumanMethylation450 BeadChip(®) for methylome profiling. PLoS One 7:e50233

36. Meissner A (2005) Reduced representation bisulfite sequencing for comparative high-resolution DNA methylation analysis. Nucleic Acids Res 33:5868–5877

37. Frommer M, McDonald LE, Millar DS et al (1992) A genomic sequencing protocol that yields a positive display of 5-methylcytosine residues in individual DNA strands. Proc Natl Acad Sci U S A 89:1827–1831

38. Grunau C, Clark SJ, Rosenthal A (2001) Bisulfite genomic sequencing: systematic investigation of critical experimental parameters. Nucleic Acids Res 29:E65–E65

39. Guo F, Yan L, Guo H et al (2015) The transcriptome and DNA methylome landscapes of human primordial germ cells. Cell 161: 1437–1452

40. Boyle P, Clement K, Gu H et al (2012) Gel-free multiplexed reduced representation bisulfite sequencing for large-scale DNA methylation profiling. Genome Biol 13:R92

41. Gu H, Bock C, Mikkelsen TS et al (2010) Genome-scale DNA methylation mapping of clinical samples at single-nucleotide resolution. Nat Methods 7:133–136

42. Smith ZD, Gu H, Bock C, Gnirke A, Meissner A (2009) High-throughput bisulfite sequencing in mammalian genomes. Methods 48:226–232

43. Liang F, Tang B, Wang Y et al (2014) WBSA: web service for bisulfite sequencing data analysis. PLoS One 9:e86707

44. Irizarry RA, Ladd-Acosta C, Wen B et al (2009) The human colon cancer methylome shows similar hypo- and hypermethylation at conserved tissue-specific CpG island shores. Nat Genet 41:178–186

45. Maunakea AK, Nagarajan RP, Bilenky M et al (2010) Conserved role of intragenic DNA methylation in regulating alternative promoters. Nature 466:253–257

46. Roessler J, Ammerpohl O, Gutwein J et al (2012) Quantitative cross-validation and content analysis of the 450k DNA methylation array from Illumina Inc. BMC Res Notes 5:210

47. Sandoval J, Heyn H, Moran S et al (2011) Validation of a DNA methylation microarray for 450,000 CpG sites in the human genome. Epigenetics 6:692–702

48. Harper KN, Peters BA, Gamble MV (2013) Batch effects and pathway analysis: two potential perils in cancer studies involving DNA methylation array analysis. Cancer Epidemiol Biomarkers Prev 22:1052–1060

49. Dedeurwaerder S, Defrance M, Calonne E, Denis H, Sotiriou C, Fuks F (2011) Evaluation of the infinium methylation 450K technology. Epigenomics 3:771–784

50. Touleimat N, Tost J (2012) Complete pipeline for Infinium(®) Human Methylation 450K BeadChip data processing using subset quantile normalization for accurate DNA methylation estimation. Epigenomics 4:325–341

51. Aryee MJ, Jaffe AE, Corrada-Bravo H et al (2014) Minfi: a flexible and comprehensive bioconductor package for the analysis of Infinium DNA methylation microarrays. Bioinformatics 30:1363–1369

52. Maksimovic J, Gordon L, Oshlack A (2012) SWAN: Subset-quantile within array normalization for illumina infinium HumanMethylation450 BeadChips. Genome Biol 13:R44

53. Teschendorff AE, Marabita F, Lechner M et al (2013) A beta-mixture quantile normalization method for correcting probe design bias in Illumina Infinium 450 k DNA methylation data. Bioinformatics 29:189–196

54. Morris TJ, Butcher LM, Feber A et al (2014) ChAMP: 450k chip analysis methylation pipeline. Bioinformatics 30:428–430

55. Pidsley R, Y Wong CC, Volta M, Lunnon K, Mill J, Schalkwyk LC (2013) A data-driven approach to preprocessing Illumina 450K methylation array data. BMC Genomics 14:293

56. Triche TJ, Weisenberger DJ, Van Den Berg D, Laird PW, Siegmund KD (2013) Low-level processing of Illumina Infinium DNA Methylation BeadArrays. Nucleic Acids Res 41:e90

57. Du P, Zhang X, Huang C-C et al (2010) Comparison of Beta-value and M-value methods for quantifying methylation levels by microarray analysis. BMC Bioinformatics 11:587

58. Bibikova M, Fan J-B (2009) GoldenGate assay for DNA methylation profiling. Methods Mol Biol 507:149–163

59. Bibikova M, Lin Z, Zhou L et al (2006) High-throughput DNA methylation profiling using universal bead arrays. Genome Res 16:383–393

60. Sean Davis, Pan Du, Sven Bilke, Tim Triche, Jr. MB. methylumi: Handle Illumina methylation data. 2015: R package version 2.14.0

61. Zhuang J, Widschwendter M, Teschendorff AE (2012) A comparison of feature selection and classification methods in DNA methylation studies using the Illumina Infinium platform. BMC Bioinformatics 13:59

62. Du P, Kibbe WA, Lin SM (2008) lumi: a pipeline for processing Illumina microarray. Bioinformatics 24:1547–1548

63. Wang D, Yan L, Hu Q et al (2012) IMA: an R package for high-throughput analysis of Illumina's 450K Infinium methylation data. Bioinformatics 28:729–730

64. Aryee KDHMJ. minfi: Analyze Illumina's 450 K methylation arrays. 2013: R package version 1.2.0. 2012

65. Butcher LM, Beck S (2015) Probe Lasso: a novel method to rope in differentially methylated regions with 450K DNA methylation data. Methods 72:21–28

66. Chen Y, Lemire M, Choufani S et al (2013) Discovery of cross-reactive probes and polymorphic CpGs in the Illumina Infinium HumanMethylation450 microarray. Epigenetics 8:203–209

Chapter 2

Reduced Representation Bisulfite Sequencing (RRBS) and Cell Sorting Prior to DNA Methylation Analysis in Psychiatric Disorders

Wilfred C. de Vega, Atif Hussain, and Patrick O. McGowan

Abstract

Gene-environment interactions play a major role in psychiatric disorder onset and manifestation. Environmental factors can influence gene expression in the absence of gene sequence alterations through epigenetic modifications such as DNA methylation at cytosine–guanine (CpG) dinucleotides. Due to decreasing costs associated with genomic sequencing, it is becoming more common to screen the DNA methylome to obtain comprehensive information regarding epigenetic modifications associated with phenotypes of interest. However, whole DNA methylome screening remains cost prohibitive and requires an intensive computational analysis. An economical alternative to screening the DNA methylome is Reduced Representation Bisulfite Sequencing (RRBS), which can be used to examine DNA methylation in CpG-dense regions at single-nucleotide resolution, thereby targeting gene regulatory elements. In this chapter, we detail the RRBS protocol, compare it to other techniques for DNA methylation sequencing, and outline its use in psychiatric genomics. We also describe Fluorescence-Activated Cell Sorting (FACS) and computational techniques that can be used to reduce variation associated with mixed cell populations in clinical samples, a potential confounding factor in epigenomics research.

Key words Psychiatric disorders, Epigenetics, Epigenomics, DNA methylation, DNA methylome, Reduced representation bisulfite sequencing, Fluorescence-activated cell sorting, Bioinformatics

1 Introduction

Psychiatric disorders are characterized by cognitive and behavioral disruptions that prevent affected individuals from carrying out their daily activities. Strong developmental origins have been observed in psychiatric disorders; however, onset tends to occur in early to late adulthood and can persist throughout life [1, 2]. Various studies have shown significant associations between genetic abnormalities and psychiatric disorders, but have not been as fruitful in explaining disease prevalence, timing, or severity as initially postulated. As with many complex diseases, the major psychiatric disorders show

Barbara Stefanska and David J. MacEwan (eds.), *Epigenetics and Gene Expression in Cancer, Inflammatory and Immune Diseases,*
Methods in Pharmacology and Toxicology, DOI 10.1007/978-1-4939-6743-8_2, © Springer Science+Business Media LLC 2017

non-Mendelian inheritance and a lack of consistent disease-specific biomarkers [3]. It is becoming increasingly recognized that gene-environment interaction also plays a prominent role in the onset and manifestation of psychiatric disorders [1, 2]. Environmental factors can interact with the genome through epigenetic modifications, which modify gene expression in the absence of gene sequence alterations. In addition to environmental factors, epigenetic differences between individuals can also occur as a function of genetic and stochastic factors [4]. One particular epigenetic mechanism that is often studied in epigenetics is DNA methylation, the addition of a methyl group on the cytosine in cytosine-guanine dinucleotide sites (CpG). In addition to DNA methylation at CpG dinucleotides, it should be noted that other forms of DNA modification exist that cannot be distinguished from DNA methylation with the methods we discuss here without procedural modifications that are beyond the scope of the present chapter. For the purposes of simplicity, then, we will use the term "DNA methylation" though DNA modification is perhaps a more appropriate descriptor.

2   Epigenetic Mechanisms in Psychiatric Disorders

Differences in DNA methylation patterns have been associated with a variety of psychiatric diseases [1, 3]. Earlier studies were often limited to a candidate gene approach. GAD67 and reelin, which are associated with cortical activity synchrony, have been implicated in schizophrenia. These genes are known to be down-regulated among individuals affected by the disease [5] and have increased DNA methylation levels in a mouse model of schizophrenia [6]. Kuratomi et al. [7] performed pyrosequencing in lymphoblastoid cells of bipolar disorder subjects and showed hypomethylation in the PPIEL gene, which corresponded to an overall mean increase in mRNA expression, drawing additional questions regarding the function of this uncharacterized gene.

More recent work on the epigenetic changes associated with psychiatric disease has begun to focus on DNA methylation differences across the genome. These studies have notably been performed with monozygotic (MZ) twins to explore why discordance in the prevalence of psychiatric disorders exists between monozygotic twins despite virtually sharing the same genome [1, 2]. Nguyen, Rauch, Pfeifer, and Hu [8] used microarray analysis and bisulfite sequencing to profile global methylation patterns of lymphoblastoid cell lines of MZ twins discordant for autism. Their study found 2 candidate genes, BCL-2 and RORA, implicated in cell death [9] and cell stress response [10], respectively, to be hypermethylated. Subsequent immunohistochemical analysis in brain tissue of autistic and age- and sex-matched controls revealed that these genes were also downregulated, linking the two levels of biological regulation together. Methylome studies have also used samples from unrelated individuals in an effort to generate candidate epigenomic loci for diagnosis using a wider population. Li et al. [11] examined the methylome in patients affected by schizophrenia or bipolar disorder and found distinct methylation differences specific to each disorder, which has implications for future biomarker research in both these diseases.

3   Reduced Representation Bisulfite Sequencing (RRBS)

Examining DNA methylation patterns across the genome can inform researchers about coordinated epigenomic differences that may underlie the disease of interest. One method that allows for methylome examination is Reduced Representation Bisulfite Sequencing (RRBS), which was developed by Meissner et al. [12]. This is accomplished by digesting the genome using a methylation-insensitive restriction enzyme, converting methylated cytosines in the short restriction fragments to uracil using sodium bisulfite, sequencing the libraries, and assembling them using bioinformatics. This method allows for the examination of particular regions of the genome that have higher CpG density, and thus maintains comprehensive coverage of the whole genome while reducing the amount of sequencing to approximately 1% of the genome [12]. In this chapter, we will compare RRBS to other methylome methods, discuss how it has been applied in neuroscience research, outline the RRBS workflow, from laboratory procedures to analytical pipelines, and discuss some limitations of this method. Following this, we will review the current issue of cell population heterogeneity in epigenetic profiling and describe how dividing cells into their distinct subpopulations using Fluorescence-Activated Cell Sorting (FACS) can help to address this particular problem.

4   Comparison of RRBS and Other Methods for Methylome Analysis

In addition to RRBS, there are multiple epigenetic profiling methods that exist. Among bisulfite sequencing methods, RRBS can be compared to Whole Genome Bisulfite Sequencing (WGBS), a bisulfite-based method that involves shotgun sequencing a bisulfite-converted DNA library. RRBS has lower sequencing depth than WGBS, where WGBS is able to provide approximately ten times more coverage of the methylome [13]. However, RRBS has been shown to have higher resolution at CpG islands, and WGBS has a greater than 50-fold increase in cost [13]. Furthermore, repeated noncoding regions of the genome are included in the final reads of WGBS, contributing to the decreased methylation mapping efficiency of WGBS and making WGBS data alignment computationally complex and expensive. Because of this, WGBS is not typically used for high-throughput methylome analysis with a large number of samples.

Currently, the most prevalent epigenetic profiling tool used in human clinical studies is the Illumina Infinium HumanMethylation450 BeadChip (450 K) array. The 450 K array provides coverage of over 99 % of RefSeq genes, while reducing the number of observations to approximately 480,000 loci across the genome [14]. The 450 K array relies on whole genome amplification and specific probe hybridization to a microarray to determine the methylation status of loci across the genome, making the array cheaper and faster than RRBS [15]. However, the costs of the next generation sequencing methods, including RRBS, have been steadily declining to the point where sequencing methods provide more data than microarrays at a comparable price [16]. In addition, RRBS requires significantly less DNA and provides higher coverage than the 450 K array [15]. Furthermore, being a sequencing-based approach, RRBS can be used on nonhuman samples, and can identify genetic mutations that overlap with methylation sites, preventing this particular confound that is observed in the 450 K array [17].

Non-bisulfite treatment-based techniques, such as Methylated DNA Immunoprecipitation Sequencing (MeDIP-seq) and Methyl-CpG Binding Domain protein sequencing (MeDIP-seq), are an alternative to bisulfite-based methods such as RRBS [18]. Contrary to RRBS, MeDIP-seq uses an anti-methylcytosine antibody to precipitate methylated DNA fragments while MBD-seq utilizes the methyl-CpG binding domain 2 (MBD2) protein to examine the methylated regions of the DNA. MeDIP-seq and MBD-seq interrogate approximately cover six times more CpGs than RRBS, which provides a better representation of the amount of methylation across the methylome. However, these techniques are more costly and are notably unable to resolve methylation differences at single-base resolution [18].

5   Application of RRBS

RRBS has been used to map methylation patterns of various organisms to create methylation reference libraries [19]. For example, Cokus et al. [20] implemented RRBS to draft the methylome of *Arabidopsis thaliana*, which was previously inaccessible due to technological constraints. The zebrafish brain methylome has also been examined with RRBS [21], demonstrating its applicability in the brain methylome research questions in model organisms. Human blood methylomes have also been generated using RRBS [22], contributing to the various human methylomes generated for the Human Methylome Project [23].

RRBS can also be used to analyze methylation patterns across different stages of development, which has notably been performed with murine embryonic stem (ES) cells. It is understood that different cell types of an organism differentiate from progenitor stem cells through the expression and silencing of particular combinations of genes [24]. In their pioneer study, Meissner et al. [12] used wild-type murine ES cells and compared them to murine ES cells that were deficient in essential DNA methylation enzymes to demonstrate the power and utility of RRBS. The study of Boyer et al. [25] also found that, on average, murine ES cells contained an increased amount of cytosine methylation relative to their differentiated cell counterparts. Spermatogenesis in murine ES cells has also been examined using RRBS [26].

Recently, RRBS has been used in clinical studies to investigate the methylation markers and patterns for neurodegenerative disorders. Liggett et al. [27] found that multiple sclerosis (MS) patients exhibit different methylation patterns relative to healthy individuals across 56 promoter regions using a microarray. Expanding on these findings, Baranzini et al. [28] implemented RRBS on four monozygotic twin pairs discordant for MS to examine genomic, methylomic, and transcriptomic changes associated with the disease. Although they did detect some epigenomic differences, the study was unable to determine a robust marker across the genomic, epigenomic, or transcriptomic levels that could explain MS discordance.

RRBS has also been used in a study by Ng et al. [29] to examine differences in Huntington's Disease, a genetic neurodegenerative disorder leading to loss of muscle control. This particular disease is caused by a CAG triplet repeat expansion, an autosomal dominant genetic mutation, in the Huntingtin gene that leads to a longer polyglutamine chain in the encoded protein [30]. Ng et al. [29] found multiple methylation differences between cell lines with a wild-type and mutated version of Huntingtin, providing additional insight on the systematic consequences of a mutated Huntingtin gene, especially at the epigenomic level.

6   RRBS: Laboratory Procedures

The principle workflow of RRBS is outlined in Fig. 1. Each major step of this protocol will be briefly outlined and summarized in a manner similar to Gu et al. [31], followed by a basic sample protocol per section.

6.1   Restriction Digest

6.1.1   Summary

DNA is first extracted and purified from the specific tissue of interest. The purity of the DNA is essential as any contaminants may affect the restriction enzyme digestion and reduce reproducibility. A restriction enzyme is added to the extracted DNA, where input

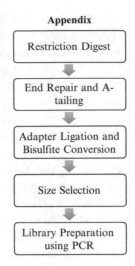

Fig. 1 Workflow of Reduced Representation Bisulfite Sequencing (RRBS)

DNA can be as little as 10 ng for digestion. Restriction enzymes must be methylation-insensitive to maximize CpG coverage of the genome and to provide reproducible fragments across RRBS libraries of difference samples. MspI is often used in RRBS as it cuts upstream of the CpG site in its recognition sequence of 3′-CCGG-5′, and restriction fragments will contain a CpG site on each end, allowing for quick identification in downstream analysis and guaranteeing at least one informative CpG read in each fragment.

6.1.2   Sample Protocol

1. Isolate DNA using the PureLink Genomic DNA kit (Invitrogen) according to the manufacturer's instructions.

2. Determine concentration of DNA using PicoGreen or a Qubit fluorometer.

3. Prepare an MspI digest using the desired amount of input DNA. A minimum of 10 ng of genomic DNA and 10 U of MspI is required.

4. Mix the reaction well and incubate at 37 °C for a minimum of 2 h.

5. To stop the reaction, add 1 μl of 0.5 M EDTA.

6. Purify the digest to remove any traces of contaminants. This can be performed using standard phenol/chloroform extraction followed by ethanol precipitation.

7. Resuspend the digested DNA in 10 mM, pH 8 Tris buffer.

6.2   End Repair and A-tailing

6.2.1   Summary

Digestion with MspI yields sticky ends that must be repaired to avoid re-annealing with nearby fragments. The overhangs are generally repaired using T4 DNA polymerase and Klenow fragments. The 3′ ends undergo A-tailing, a procedure that adds an extra single adenosine nucleotide originating from dATP. The resulting

A-tail serves to facilitate subsequent adapter ligation to the ends of the fragments.

6.2.2 Sample Protocol

1. Repair and A-tail the digested DNA using T4 DNA polymerase, Klenow fragments, and deoxynucleotides. For A-tailing to be successful, the concentration of dATP must be 10× greater relative to the other deoxynucleotides.

2. Mix reaction well and incubate at 20 °C for 20 min (end repair) followed by a 37 °C incubation step for 20 min (A-tailing).

3. Purify the reaction as previously described.

6.3 Adapter Ligation and Bisulfite Conversion

6.3.1 Summary

Once the DNA has been repaired, an adapter must be attached onto each fragment to allow for PCR amplification in later steps in the workflow. The adapter is typically from Illumina and is 60 bp in length with 5'-methylated cytosines. These methylated cytosines will resist deamination during bisulfite conversion and serve as an internal control in downstream bioinformatics analysis. Either standard- or paired-end adapters can be used depending on the type of study; however, paired-end adapters can provide greater coverage for regions beside the restriction sites such as CpG island shores [31]. The DNA is then treated with sodium bisulfite, which converts unmethylated cytosines to uracil while methylated cytosines will remain unaffected [12]. In subsequent PCR steps of the bisulfite conversion protocol, unmethylated cytosines will be represented with thymidines as a result of the uracil replacement.

6.3.2 Sample Protocol

1. Prepare the ligation reaction with Illumina adapters and T4 DNA ligase. Methylated adapters should be added at a minimum final working concentration of 0.75 μM.

2. Mix the reaction well and incubate at 16 °C overnight (16–24 h).

3. Purify the DNA as previously described.

4. Perform bisulfite conversion on the ligated DNA and purify the DNA as previously described.

6.4 Size Selection

6.4.1 Summary

Size selection is performed to obtain the optimal fragments for genome coverage and to remove restriction fragments that failed to ligate with the adapters. This is typically achieved by cutting out portions of a 1.5–3 % gel corresponding to the size range of interest after running the restriction fragments on the gel. Inserts within the size range of 40–220 bp adequately represent the majority of CpG islands and promoter regions across the genome.

6.4.2 Sample Protocol

1. Prepare a low melt agarose gel (Nusieve) at the desired concentration (1.5–3 %).

2. Load samples into gel, ensuring that three lanes separate each sample to prevent any bleed over.

3. Run the gel at 5 V/cm until the loading dye marker is 6–7 cm away from the wells.

4. If single-end reads will be performed, excise 160–400 bp from the gel. If paired-end reads will be performed, excise 170–410 bp from the gel.

5. Extract the DNA using a gel extraction kit (Qiagen MinElute Gel Extraction Kit) and purify the DNA.

6.5 Library Preparation Using PCR

6.5.1 Summary

In order to reduce PCR bias, a small amount of the extracted DNA can be run for a test PCR using various cycles to determine the minimum number of cycles to produce an evenly represented library. Quantitative real-time PCR (qPCR) can also be used to determine the threshold cycle. Afterward, the library is prepared by running PCR on the excised DNA with the predetermined number of cycles. The library is purified using AMPure XP magnetic beads. A final quality control check is typically performed to ensure the library is free of contaminants and of adapters that did not ligate to any restriction fragments.

6.5.2 Sample Protocol

1. Using primers complementary to the Illumina adapters and a small amount of extract DNA, perform qPCR to determine the threshold cycle.

2. Once the threshold cycle is determined, perform PCR using the same primers and with the predetermined amount of cycles. An example of a PCR protocol would be: 1 cycle of 45 s @ 98 °C, cycles of 15 s @ 98 °C, 30 s @ 60 °C, and 30 s @ 72 °C (number of cycles depends on qPCR results), and 1 final cycle of 1 min @ 72 °C.

3. Transfer PCR products to a fresh tube and mix with a manufacturer-recommended amount of room temperature AMPure XP beads.

4. Incubate mixture at room temperature for 15 min.

5. Insert tube into DynaMag-2 magnet for 5–10 min.

6. Remove aqueous phase and add 1 ml of 70% (v/v) ethanol without interrupting magnetic beads.

7. Incubate mixture for 5 min.

8. Repeat Steps 6 and 7 to perform a second wash of the beads.

9. Remove aqueous phase and let beads air dry from up to 5 min.

10. Remove tube from magnet and resuspend beads with Tris buffer.

11. Place tube back to a magnet to separate the beads from the DNA.

12. Carefully remove the DNA solution without disturbing the beads and transfer to a new tube.

13. Verify the quality of the library using a polyacrylamide gel to ensure no contaminants are present. A Bioanalyzer gel can also be used to examine the banding pattern of the library.

14. If the library fails the quality control check or there are adapters present in the library, repeat the Size Selection step and re-purify the DNA using AMPure XP magnetic beads.

7 RRBS: Sequencing and Analysis

The RRBS library is then sequenced to determine the methylation status of various CpG loci across the genome. Sequencing is typically performed using next generation sequencing methods such as Illumina HiSeq. As previously stated, proper MspI digestion will produce fragments with a CpG site flanking both sites, and will allow for better identification of informative reads by searching for this particular pattern. Platforms such as the Illumina HiSeq produce 30–40 million reads per sample [31, 32].

Preparing sequenced library data for analysis typically requires multiple computing languages and an adept working knowledge of bioinformatics coding. Sequences are first trimmed from their adapters in silico using analytical packages such as Trim Galore (http://www.bioinformatics.babraham.ac.uk/projects/trim_galore/). The trimmed sequences are then aligned to the genome using available bioinformatics packages such as Bowtie [33] or custom software developed for RRBS [31, 34]. Methylation calls are then typically made using packages such as Bismark [35] and MethylKit [36]. Identifying differentially methylated regions can be accomplished by comparing the differences in reads between the experimental and control samples.

8 Limitations of RRBS

RRBS has notable advantages over other methylome techniques, and also some limitations. Restriction digestion with MspI will bias results toward CpG-rich regions, providing high coverage for promoter regions and most CpG islands but little to no coverage for CpG-poor regions. This is a major limitation of RRBS for researchers seeking to examine DNA methylation differences comprehensively across specific genomic loci. It is recommended that an in silico analysis is performed prior to performing RRBS to ensure the region of interest has sufficient coverage for analytical purposes [31].

The efficiency of bisulfite conversion and degradation of DNA are also concerns since harsh conditions are implemented and a non-proofreading Taq polymerase is used to prevent stalling at uracil bases during PCR amplification. If the template DNA is not completely denatured, incomplete bisulfite conversion may occur, introducing experimental artifacts that may confound true methylation status. However, the higher temperatures that are used to ensure complete denaturation may lead to DNA degradation, which further hinders the PCR amplification process and may introduce additional errors in the library preparation. Meissner et al. [12] addressed this concern by including urea during bisulfite conversion and carefully optimizing the PCR protocol to minimize PCR bias and DNA degradation.

9   Cell Type Selection, Heterogeneity, and Its Effect on Epigenomic Data

Ideally in the context of psychiatric disorders, neurons would be the tissue of choice, as it would best inform researchers of dysregulation in the brain. A number of studies have examined the specific neuronal differences associated with psychiatric disorders in rodent models and human subjects [37]. Of course, the obvious limitations to this approach are that it is not possible to identify brain-specific biomarkers for clinical diagnosis and to track differences over the progression of the disorder since brain tissue is not available for sampling in living humans. An alternative to this approach is to examine peripheral tissue such as blood and saliva, which are highly accessible and use noninvasive methods for acquisition. Indeed, many studies have been undertaken to understand how differences in the brain are reflected in the periphery [37–39].

Some genes that were found to be differentially regulated in psychiatric disorders by examining postmortem brain tissue also show differential methylation in peripheral tissues among living individuals [40]. BDNF has been found to be differentially methylated in peripheral blood of patients who suffer from major depression [41]. Oberlander et al. [42] found DNA methylation differences in NR3C1 of cord blood from infants of depressed mothers, which were reflected in salivary cortisol differences. Notably, however, for biomarker discovery it is not necessary that the differential methylation be identical to that identified in neural tissue for the biomarker to serve a useful diagnostic purpose.

While RRBS allows for the visualization of genome-wide methylation patterns, it is important to note that every cell type has, to some extent, its own unique epigenomic signature [23]. Thus, it is becoming increasingly recognized that DNA methylation differences detected in studies that utilize mixed cell populations such as blood and brain tissue may be confounded due to cell type composition differences [43]. One method that directly addresses this issue is to perform FACS on mixed cell populations and separate them into their respective cell populations using antibodies for the populations of interest. Epigenomic assays can then be performed on these separated fractions without the issue of cell population heterogeneity.

This particular method has been implemented in studies examining brain and blood. Iwamoto et al. [44] separated neuronal and non-neuronal cells from human prefrontal cortex samples using a NeuN antibody, an established marker for neurons, and examined methylome differences using the luminometric methylation assay method and the Illumina GoldenGate assay. There were distinct differences between neuronal cells and non-neuronal cells where neurons showed global hypomethylation, greater DNA methylation variation, and increased methylation in genes typically expressed in astrocytes. Reinius et al. [45] also implemented FACS to sort whole human blood into seven different subpopulations and used the 450 K array to probe methylome differences. Different DNA methylation patterns emerged for each subpopulation, underlining the unique methylome signatures found in distinct blood cell populations and the need to exercise caution when interpreting epigenomic results from whole blood studies.

10 FACS: Laboratory Procedures

The principle workflow of FACS is outlined in Fig. 2. Each step will be outlined and summarized, followed by a basic protocol when required.

10.1 Antibody Selection

10.1.1 Summary

Prior to performing FACS, it is imperative that the appropriate antibodies are selected for the cell population of interest. Common antibodies include NeuN for neuronal cells, CD3 for T cells, CD19 for B cells, and CD56 for NK cells. Depending on the cell population of interest, more than one antibody may be required, which can possibly affect future steps of the FACS protocol. An example of this is CD4 T cells, which require both CD3 and CD4 antibodies to be correctly sorted into its own individual subpopulation. Fluorophores are also important to consider when selecting

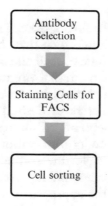

Fig. 2 Workflow of Fluorescence Activated Cell Sorting (FACS)

antibodies as this will determine the types of lasers that will be used in the FACS sorter. Fluorophores with conflicting wavelengths will hinder the ability of the sorter to accurately sort the cells; therefore, it is recommended to consult with an antibody manufacturer or an experienced FACS technician to select the best and appropriate fluorophores for the experiment.

10.2 Staining Cells for FACS

10.2.1 Summary

Cells must be stained with the antibodies before being placed in a FACS sorter. A cell viability marker such as DAPI is usually added to sort for live cells since dead cells may contaminate the sorted cell populations. Avoid light exposure as much as possible to retain the strongest possible signal from the fluorophores. If working with cryopreserved samples, rapid thawing in a water bath is required to maintain cell viability for the experiment prior to staining. Washing cryopreserved cells is also essential to remove any residual DMSO that may affect cell viability.

10.2.2 Sample Protocol

1. Place desired number of cells into 96-well V-bottomed plates.
2. Centrifuge plates at $200 \times g$ for 10 min to pellet the cells.
3. Remove the supernatant and resuspend cells in PBS+0.1% NaN_3 +0.5% bovine serum albumin.
4. Add the appropriate antibody panels and cell viability markers as recommended by the manufacturer.
5. Incubate cells with the markers in the dark at 4 °C for 30 min.
6. Centrifuge plates at $200 \times g$ for 10 min and remove the supernatant.
7. Wash cells by resuspending in PBS+0.1% NaN_3 +0.5% BSA.
8. Repeat **steps 6** and **7** for an additional wash step.
9. Fix cells with 200 µl of PBS +2% paraformaldehyde.
10. Store plates at 4 °C in the dark until ready for sorting. Process samples within 24 h of staining to maintain strong signals from the fluorophores.

10.3 Cell Sorting

10.3.1 Summary

In FACS, the cell suspension is passed through a narrow stream of liquid such that the timing between each cell allows for sufficient time to read and sort according to the predetermined parameters. An internal vibration mechanism separates each cell into individual droplets and cells flow through one at a time in the stream. Lasers of desired wavelengths are then used to determine the amount of fluorescence and light scatter properties of the cell under observation. Forward scatter indicates the size of the cell while side scatter reveals cell granularity. Based on the fluorescence and light scatter properties of the cell, the cell is sorted into the appropriate bin, according to the gates implemented by the user, by applying different electric charges to move the cell into the appropriate container.

The number of cell populations that can be collected will depend on the cell sorter, but typically 2–6 subpopulations are acquired from a FACS run. In order to determine the appropriate gates and electric settings to sort the cell populations of interest, it is recommended to consult the antibody manufacturer's recommendations of or an experienced FACS technician to ensure accurate cell sorting.

11   Computational Alternative to Cell Sorting

While FACS is a well-validated method to separate cell populations, it is sometimes not feasible to perform, as it is a laborious method that cannot be performed in a high-throughput manner. This issue has been recently addressed through computational methods in blood samples. Houseman et al. [43] produced an algorithm that corrects for cell heterogeneity in a given dataset by comparing the methylation profile of loci that are characteristic of specific blood cell populations such as T cells, B cells, and granulocytes. By using the methylation signatures for each cell type, this method attempts to correct for cell type heterogeneity and remove methylation differences that were due to differences in cell proportion. Zou et al. [46] also created a new algorithm that corrects for heterogeneity without requiring prior knowledge of the cell populations present in the sample. The use of surrogate variables can allow researchers to correct epigenomic data on non-blood tissues; however, to our knowledge, there have been no epigenomic studies in brain tissue that have used reliable computational methods to correct for cell proportion prior to methylome analysis.

12   Conclusion

The application of RRBS alongside cell sorting could be conducive to a new understanding of epigenetic mechanisms in psychiatric disorders. Schizophrenia, bipolar disorder, and autism are examples of psychiatric disorders that have been previously associated with methylation pattern differences. This technique allows researchers to understand genome-wide methylation patterns with single-base resolution, which adds to the growing amount of available methylome data associated with these diseases.

Unlike genetic aberrations, epigenetic changes are potentially reversible, providing the possibility of targeted epigenetic therapies through pharmaceutical intervention [2]. Pharmaceutical intervention has been examined in some drugs that have document epigenomic activity. Chronically stressed mice that exhibit depressive-like symptoms have decreases in histone H3K14 acetylation levels in the nucleus accumbens [47]. Pena and colleagues treated these mice with fluoxetine, a commonly prescribed antidepressant with known histone modification activity, and found that treatment with fluoextine increased histone acetylation to control levels. Similarly, research in models of multiple sclerosis have focused on the benefits of using histone deacetylase inhibitors such as valproic acid, to downregulate and reduce the impact of MECP2 expression in the hopes of finding a potential cure to the disease [48]. The application of RRBS in psychiatric disorder research provides a relatively cost-effective methylation analysis tool to contribute to a growing understanding of epigenome-wide differences in DNA methylation associated with psychiatric disease and the biological systems dysregulated in these disorders and are of great benefit especially in clinical research contexts.

13 Appendix

References

1. Ptak C, Petronis A (2010) Epigenetic approaches to psychiatric disorders. Dialogues Clin Neurosci 12(1):25–35

2. Sasaki A, de Vega WC, McGowan PO (2013) Biological embedding in mental health: an epigenomic perspective. Biochem Cell Biol 91(1):14–21

3. Grayson DR, Guidotti A (2013) The dynamics of DNA methylation in schizophrenia and related psychiatric disorders. Neuropsychopharmacology 38(1):138–166

4. Petronis A (2010) Epigenetics as a unifying principle in the aetiology of complex traits and diseases. Nature 465(7299):721–727

5. Gavin DP, Sharma RP (2010) Histone modifications, DNA methylation, and schizophrenia. Neurosci Biobehav Rev 34(6):882–888

6. Guidotti A, Auta J, Chen Y, Davis JM, Dong E, Gavin DP, Grayson DR, Matrisciano F, Pinna G, Satta R, Sharma RP, Tremolizzo L, Tueting P (2011) Epigenetic GABAergic targets in schizophrenia and bipolar disorder. Neuropharmacology 60(7-8):1007–1016

7. Kuratomi G, Iwamoto K, Bundo M, Kusumi I, Kato N, Iwata N, Ozaki N, Kato T (2008) Aberrant DNA methylation associated with bipolar disorder identified from discordant monozygotic twins. Mol Psychiatry 13(4):429–441

8. Nguyen A, Rauch TA, Pfeifer GP, Hu VW (2010) Global methylation profiling of lymphoblastoid cell lines reveals epigenetic contributions to autism spectrum disorders and a novel autism candidate gene, RORA, whose protein product is reduced in autistic brain. FASEB J 24(8):3036–3051

9. Hockenbery D, Nunez G, Milliman C, Schreiber RD, Korsmeyer SJ (1990) Bcl-2 is an inner mitochondrial membrane protein that blocks programmed cell death. Nature 348(6299):334–336. doi:10.1038/348334a0

10. Zhu Y, McAvoy S, Kuhn R, Smith DI (2006) RORA, a large common fragile site gene, is involved in cellular stress response. Oncogene 25(20):2901–2908. doi:10.1038/sj.onc.1209314

11. Li Y, Camarillo C, Xu J, Arana TB, Xiao Y, Zhao Z, Chen H, Ramirez M, Zavala J, Escamilla MA, Armas R, Mendoza R, Ontiveros A, Nicolini H, Magaña AA, Rubin LP, Li X, Xu C (2015) Genome-wide methylome analyses reveal novel epigenetic regulation patterns in schizophrenia and bipolar disorder. Biomed Res Int 2015:201587

12. Meissner A, Gnirke A, Bell GW, Ramsahoye B, Lander ES, Jaenisch R (2005) Reduced representation bisulfite sequencing for comparative high-resolution DNA methylation analysis. Nucleic Acids Res 33(18):5868–5877

13. Doherty R, Couldrey C (2014) Exploring genome wide bisulfite sequencing for DNA methylation analysis in livestock: a technical assessment. Front Genet 5:126

14. Bibikova M, Barnes B, Tsan C, Ho V, Klotzle B, Le JM, Delano D, Zhang L, Schroth GP, Gunderson KL, Fan JB, Shen R (2011) High density DNA methylation array with single CpG site resolution. Genomics 98(4):288–295

15. Pan H, Chen L, Dogra S, Teh AL, Tan JH, Lim YI, Lim YC, Jin S, Lee YK, Ng PY, Ong ML, Barton S, Chong YS, Meaney MJ,

Gluckman PD, Stunkel W, Ding C, Holbrook JD (2012) Measuring the methylome in clinical samples: improved processing of the Infinium Human Methylation450 BeadChip Array. Epigenetics 7(10):1173–1187

16. Huang YW, Huang TH, Wang LS (2010) Profiling DNA methylomes from microarray to genome-scale sequencing. Technol Cancer Res Treat 9(2):139–147

17. Chen YA, Lemire M, Choufani S, Butcher DT, Grafodatskaya D, Zanke BW, Gallinger S, Hudson TJ, Weksberg R (2013) Discovery of cross-reactive probes and polymorphic CpGs in the Illumina Infinium HumanMethylation450 microarray. Epigenetics 8(2):203–209

18. Harris RA, Wang T, Coarfa C, Nagarajan RP, Hong C, Downey SL, Johnson BE, Fouse SD, Delaney A, Zhao Y, Olshen A, Ballinger T, Zhou X, Forsberg KJ, Gu J, Echipare L, O'Geen H, Lister R, Pelizzola M, Xi Y, Epstein CB, Bernstein BE, Hawkins RD, Ren B, Chung WY, Gu H, Bock C, Gnirke A, Zhang MQ, Haussler D, Ecker JR, Li W, Farnham PJ, Waterland RA, Meissner A, Marra MA, Hirst M, Milosavljevic A, Costello JF (2010) Comparison of sequencing-based methods to profile DNA methylation and identification of monoallelic epigenetic modifications. Nat Biotechnol 28(10):1097–1105

19. Smith ZD, Gu H, Bock C, Gallinger S, Meissner A (2009) High-throughput bisulfite sequencing in mammalian genomes. Methods 48(3):226–232

20. Cokus SJ, Feng S, Zhang X, Chen Z, Merriman B, Haudenschild CD, Pradhan S, Nelson SF, Pellegrini M, Jacobsen SE (2008) Shotgun bisulphite sequencing of the Arabidopsis genome reveals DNA methylation patterning. Nature 452(7184):215–219. doi:10.1038/nature06745

21. Chatterjee A, Ozaki Y, Stockwell PA, Horsfield JA, Morison IM, Nakagawa S (2013) Mapping the zebrafish brain methylome using reduced representation bisulfite sequencing. Epigenetics 8(9):979–989

22. Wang L, Sun J, Wu H, Liu S, Wang J, Wu B, Huang S, Li N, Wang J, Zhang X (2012) Systematic assessment of reduced representation bisulfite sequencing to human blood samples: A promising method for large-sample-scale epigenomic studies. J Biotechnol 157(1):1–6

23. Kundaje A, Meuleman W, Ernst J, Bilenky M, Yen A, Heravi-Moussavi A, Kheradpour P, Zhang Z, Wang J, Ziller MJ, Amin V, Whitaker JW, Schultz MD, Ward LD, Sarkar A, Quon G, Sandstrom RS, Eaton ML, Wu YC, Pfenning AR, Wang X, Claussnitzer M, Liu Y, Coarfa C, Harris RA, Shoresh N, Epstein CB, Gjoneska E, Leung D, Xie W, Hawkins RD, Lister R, Hong C, Gascard P, Mungall AJ, Moore R, Chuah E, Tam A, Canfield TK, Hansen RS, Kaul R, Sabo PJ, Bansal MS, Carles A, Dixon JR, Farh KH, Feizi S, Karlic R, Kim AR, Kulkarni A, Li D, Lowdon R, Elliott G, Mercer TR, Neph SJ, Onuchic V, Polak P, Rajagopal N, Ray P, Sallari RC, Siebenthall KT, Sinnott-Armstrong NA, Stevens M, Thurman RE, Wu J, Zhang B, Zhou X, Beaudet AE, Boyer LA, De Jager PL, Farnham PJ, Fisher SJ, Haussler D, Jones SJ, Li W, Marra MA, McManus MT, Sunyaev S, Thomson JA, Tlsty TD, Tsai LH, Wang W, Waterland RA, Zhang MQ, Chadwick LH, Bernstein BE, Costello JF, Ecker JR, Hirst M, Meissner A, Milosavljevic A, Ren B, Stamatoyannopoulos JA, Wang T, Kellis M, Roadmap Epigenomics Consortium (2015) Integrative analysis of 111 reference human epigenomes. Nature 518(7539):317–330

24. Keller GM (1995) In vitro differentiation of embryonic stem cells. Curr Opin Cell Biol 7(6):862–869

25. Boyer LA, Plath K, Zeitlinger J, Brambrink T, Medeiros LA, Lee TI, Levine SS, Wernig M, Tajonar A, Ray MK, Bell GW, Otte AP, Vidal M, Gifford DK, Young RA, Jaenisch R (2006) Polycomb complexes repress developmental regulators in murine embryonic stem cells. Nature 441(7091):349–353. doi:10.1038/nature04733

26. Guo H, Zhu P, Wu X, Li X, Wen L, Tang F (2013) Single-cell methylome landscapes of mouse embryonic stem cells and early embryos analyzed using reduced representation bisulfite sequencing. Genome Res 23(12):2126–2135. doi:10.1101/gr.161679.113

27. Liggett T, Melnikov A, Tilwalli S, Yi Q, Chen H, Replogle C, Feng X, Reder A, Stefoski D, Balabanov R, Levenson V (2010) Methylation patterns of cell-free plasma DNA in relapsing-remitting multiple sclerosis. J Neurol Sci 290(1-2):16–21

28. Baranzini SE, Mudge J, van Velkinburgh JC, Khankhanian P, Khrebtukova I, Miller NA, Zhang L, Farmer AD, Bell CJ, Kim RW, May GD, Woodward JE, Caillier SJ, McElroy JP, Gomez R, Pando MJ, Clendenen LE, Ganusova EE, Schilkey FD, Ramaraj T, Khan OA, Huntley JJ, Luo S, Kwok PY, Wu TD, Schroth GP, Oksenberg JR, Hauser SL, Kingsmore SF (2010) Genome, epigenome and RNA sequences of monozygotic twins discordant for multiple sclerosis. Nature 464(7293):1351–1356

29. Ng CW, Yildirim F, Yap YS, Dalin S, Matthews BJ, Velez PJ, Labadorf A, Housman DE, Fraenkel E (2013) Extensive changes in DNA methylation are associated with expression of mutant huntingtin. Proc Natl Acad Sci U S A 110(6):2354–2359

30. Landles C, Bates GP (2004) Huntingtin and the molecular pathogenesis of Huntington's disease. Fourth in molecular medicine review series. EMBO Rep 5(10):958–963

31. Gu H, Smith ZD, Bock C, Boyle P, Gnirke A, Meissner A (2011) Preparation of reduced representation bisulfite sequencing libraries for genome-scale DNA methylation profiling. Nat Protoc 6(4):468–481

32. Bock C, Tomazou EM, Brinkman AB, Müller F, Simmer F, Gu H, Jäger N, Gnirke A, Stunnenberg HG, Meissner A (2010) Quantitative comparison of genome-wide DNA methylation mapping technologies. Nat Biotechnol 28(10):1106–1114

33. Langmead B, Salzberg SL (2012) Fast gapped-read alignment with Bowtie 2. Nat Methods 9(4):357–359. doi:10.1038/nmeth.1923

34. Meissner A, Mikkelsen TS, Gu H, Wernig M, Hanna J, Sivachenko A, Zhang X, Bernstein BE, Nusbaum C, Jaffe DB, Gnirke A, Jaenisch R, Lander ES (2008) Genome-scale DNA methylation maps of pluripotent and differentiated cells. Nature 454(7205):766–770

35. Krueger F, Andrews SR (2011) Bismark: a flexible aligner and methylation caller for Bisulfite-Seq applications. Bioinformatics 27(11):1571–1572. doi:10.1093/bioinformatics/btr167

36. Akalin A, Kormaksson M, Li S, Garrett-Bakelman FE, Figueroa ME, Melnick A, Mason CE (2012) methylKit: a comprehensive R package for the analysis of genome-wide DNA methylation profiles. Genome Biol 13(10):R87. doi:10.1186/gb-2012-13-10-r87

37. Tsankova N, Renthal W, Kumar A, Nestler EJ (2007) Epigenetic regulation in psychiatric disorders. Nat Rev Neurosci 8(5):355–367

38. Chrousos GP (2009) Stress and disorders of the stress system. Nat Rev Endocrinol 5(7):374–381

39. Pariante CM, Lightman SL (2008) The HPA axis in major depression: classical theories and new developments. Trends Neurosci 31(9):464–468

40. Klengel T, Pape J, Binder EB, Mehta D (2014) The role of DNA methylation in stress-related psychiatric disorders. Neuropharmacology 80:115–132

41. Fuchikami M, Morinobu S, Segawa M, Okamoto Y, Yamawaki S, Ozaki N, Inoue T, Kusumi I, Koyama T, Tsuchiyama K, Terao T (2011) DNA methylation profiles of the brain-derived neurotrophic factor (BDNF) gene as a potent diagnostic biomarker in major depression. PLoS One 6(8):e23881

42. Oberlander TF, Weinberg J, Papsdorf M, Grunau R, Misri S, Devlin AM (2008) Prenatal exposure to maternal depression, neonatal methylation of human glucocorticoid receptor gene (NR3C1) and infant cortisol stress responses. Epigenetics 3(2):97–106

43. Houseman EA, Accomando WP, Koestler DC, Christensen BC, Marsit CJ, Nelson HH, Wiencke JK, Kelsey KT (2012) DNA methylation arrays as surrogate measures of cell mixture distribution. BMC Bioinformatics 13:86

44. Iwamoto K, Bundo M, Ueda J, Oldham MC, Ukai W, Hashimoto E, Saito T, Geschwind DH, Kato T (2011) Neurons show distinctive DNA methylation profile and higher interindividual variations compared with non-neurons. Genome Res 21(5):688–696

45. Reinius LE, Acevedo N, Joerink M, Pershagen G, Dahlén SE, Greco D, Söderhäll C, Scheynius A, Kere J (2012) Differential DNA methylation in purified human blood cells: implications for cell lineage and studies on disease susceptibility. PLoS One 7(7):e41361

46. Zou J, Lippert C, Heckerman D, Aryee M, Listgarten J (2014) Epigenome-wide association studies without the need for cell-type composition. Nat Methods 11(3):309–311

47. Pena CJ, Bagot RC, Labonte B, Nestler EJ (2014) Epigenetic signaling in psychiatric disorders. J Mol Biol 426(20):3389–3412. doi:10.1016/j.jmb.2014.03.016

48. KhorshidAhmad T, Acosta C, Cortes C, Lakowski TM, Gangadaran S, Namaka M (2015) Transcriptional Regulation of Brain-Derived Neurotrophic Factor (BDNF) by Methyl CpG Binding Protein 2 (MeCP2): a Novel Mechanism for Re-Myelination and/or Myelin Repair Involved in the Treatment of Multiple Sclerosis (MS)., Mol Neurobiol

Chapter 3

Targeted DNA Methylation Analysis Methods

David Cheishvili, Sophie Petropoulos, Steffan Christiansen, and Moshe Szyf

Abstract

DNA methylation is an important enzymatic covalent modification of DNA that plays an important role in genome regulation. DNA methylation patterns are fashioned during development and could be altered in response to experience and exposure. Aberrations in DNA methylation patterns are noted in cancer and other diseases. It is therefore extremely important to accurately quantify DNA methylation states for studying physiology and disease as well as for using DNA methylation markers in diagnosis. Here, we review the most commonly used methods for quantifying DNA methylation states of single genes: Pyrosequencing, Quantitative Methylated DNA Immunoprecipitation (qMeDIP), and methylation-sensitive high resolution melting (MS-HRM). Each method is described and required steps are detailed. We also discuss the advantages and disadvantages of the different methods.

Key words DNA methylation, Sodium bisulfite, Quantitative Methylated DNA Immunoprecipitation (qMeDIP), Methylation-sensitive high resolution melting (MS-HRM), Pyrosequencing

Abbreviations

dsDNA double-stranded DNA
FFPE Formalin-fixed paraffin-embedded tissue
GWAS Genome-Wide Association Study
MeDIP methylated DNA immunoprecipitation
RRBS Reduced representation bisulfite sequencing

1 Introduction

Recent advances in DNA sequencing technology have led to a significant reduction in the cost of genome wide analysis, which in turn has increased the number of genome-wide association studies (GWAS). Though the data obtained from high-through-put genome-wide experimental approaches (MeDIP-seq/ChIP,

Barbara Stefanska and David J. MacEwan (eds.), *Epigenetics and Gene Expression in Cancer, Inflammatory and Immune Diseases,* Methods in Pharmacology and Toxicology, DOI 10.1007/978-1-4939-6743-8_3, © Springer Science+Business Media LLC 2017

RRBS, and Illumina 450 K), as discussed in Chap. 1 entitled "High-Troughput Techniques for DNA Methylation Profiling" are of significant analytical value, downstream experimental validation and refining of the data generated is required. For such purposes, targeted methods of DNA methylation are utilized.

When choosing the targeted method of analysis, available expertise, financial means, and equipment limitations within the laboratory are usually taken into consideration first of all. It should be noted however that this approach is not always justified in the long run.

While choosing the method one should consider the technical characteristics such as size of DNA fragment to be amplified and its complexity, limitations and advantages of each technique, time required for the method, and the aim of the experiment. A number of methods are available for targeted DNA methylation assessment: bisulfite sequencing, quantitative methylated DNA immunoprecipitation (qMeDIP), pyrosequencing [1], methylation-sensitive high resolution melting (MS-HRM) [2], and combined bisulfite restriction analysis (COBRA) [3].

For many years, bisulfite sequencing has served as the "gold standard" for measuring DNA methylation. However, this procedure is cumbersome, expensive and the results are based on analysis of approximately 10–20 colonies, which is often considered underpowered, thus making it difficult to obtain statistically meaningful results. Methods with improved quantitative resolution such as pyrosequencing, MS-HRM, and qMeDIP are effective alternatives. In this chapter, the pros and cons of these most commonly used targeted approaches will be discussed.

2   DNA Methylation Analysis by Pyrosequencing

2.1   Pyrosequencing Overview

Pyrosequencing is a real-time DNA sequencing-by-synthesis method, which was developed by Mostafa Ronaghi and Pal Nyren at the Royal Institute of Technology in 1996 [4]. The development of this technique evolved due to the need for a method that would address deficiencies in established bisulfite sequencing methods (discussed later).

Its ease of use, high reliability, flexibility, and efficiency has made pyrosequencing a widely used platform for various diagnostic applications such as genotyping [5] and mutations detection [6]. Here, we will discuss pyrosequencing application in DNA methylation assessment.

Pyrosequencing is a DNA sequencing technique that relies on the bioluminometric detection of pyrophosphate release upon the introduction of a nucleotide [4, 7] and uses a single biotinylated primer that is incorporated into PCR product during amplification reaction. This is in contrast to the Sanger method, which is based on selective incorporation of one of four fluorescently labeled terminating dideoxynucleotides (ddNTPs) during DNA polymerase mediated in vitro replication [8]. Further, in comparison to Sanger sequencing, pyrosequencing can assess DNA methylation with greater efficiency. In pyrosequencing a single reaction can sequence hundreds or thousands of different DNA molecules at once, allowing the assessment of methylation for thousands of DNA copies. Moreover, while bisulfite sequencing requires multiple steps, pyrosequencing requires two steps: PCR amplification followed by pyrosequencing itself. A disadvantage of pyrosequencing is the shorter length of the sequence read (25-100 bp) in comparison with bisulfite sequencing (~500 bp). However this limitation can be partially overcome by the use of the same template several times with staggered sequencing primers.

Pyrosequencing includes the following steps:

- DNA extraction and bisulfite conversion.

- Assay and primers design.

- PCR of bisulfite-treated DNA.

- Pyrosequencing, that measures DNA methylation at a single nucleotide resolution within the region of interest.

- Data analysis.

2.2 Genomic DNA Preparation and DNA Concentration Measurement

The quality of extracted DNA is a very important factor that may affect further bisulfite conversion efficiency. Degraded starting material will lead to increased sample loss during the bisulfite conversion process. To obtain high quality, RNA, and protein free genomic DNA one can choose between the multitude of commercially available spin-column-based assays, which provide custom kits depending on the source of sample (i.e., human or animal tissue, cultured cells, cultured bacteria, formalin-fixed paraffin-embedded tissue (FFPE) sections, blood, plants, etc.). Alternatively, in-house extraction protocols can also be used comprising of a lysis buffer followed by phenol–chloroform DNA isolation and precipitated with 95 % (v/v) ethanol [9, 10]. One of the critical steps prior to phenol/chloroform DNA extraction is Proteinase K treatment. Proteinase K treatment digests contaminating proteins, which includes chromatin associated with DNA; the presence of which can hinder the dissociation reaction of the two DNA strands. In addition, Proteinase K digests nucleases that can degrade nucleic acid [11].

Following DNA isolation, measurement of both the quantity and quality is required. An accurate measurement of DNA concentration is critical to the success of efficient bisulfite conversion and further DNA methylation assessment. Variability in genomic DNA concentrations when comparing two different samples may affect interpretation of DNA methylation results. There are numerous methods that can be used to measure quantity of the genomic DNA, such as UV spectroscopy (regular spectrophotometers or more advanced, Nanodrop) and Fluorometric analysis (PicoGreen® and Qubit®). Measurements of DNA concentration with Fluorometric methods (Qubit able to quantitate from 10 pg/µL up to 1 µg/µL and PicoGreen-able to quantitate from 25 pg/mL up to 100 ng/mL of dsDNA), which are based on target-specific fluorescent dyes, are preferred over using an optical density spectrophotometric method (UV spectroscopy), which does not distinguish between DNA, RNA, protein, free nucleotides, or amino acids in the sample and often leads to over-estimation of the DNA concentration. In addition, the spectrophotometric method is influenced by a variety of biomolecules as well as dust particles [12–15]. Spectrometric methods, however, can be used to measure UV absorbance ratios for DNA purity (260/280 UV) and other contaminants (260/230 UV), where ratios of ~1.8 and 2.0–2.2, respectively, are considered ideal.

Finally, visualization of genomic DNA by agarose gel electrophoresis to assess integrity is recommended. A high molecular weight band should be visible as opposed to smears, which would indicate degradation of DNA.

2.3 DNA Bisulfite Treatment

DNA methylation analysis in pyrosequencing as well as MS-HRM starts with bisulfite treatment of genomic DNA. Since the original discovery in 1970 [16, 17], DNA bisulfite conversion has become the most popular tool to investigate DNA methylation [18]. DNA bisulfite conversion is based on the ability of sulfite to be reversibly added to cytosine to mediate the deamination of unmethylated cytosine to uracil. However, when the cytosine is methylated, deamination reaction is prevented and cytosine remains unaffected. The critical step in the conversion process is denaturation of the double-stranded DNA prior to conversion, since only cytosine in single-stranded DNA molecules is deaminated. Failure of the denaturation step can lead to artifacts and incomplete conversion of DNA and ultimately misinterpretation of the final data. Strong bias was reported previously [19] toward amplification of unmethylated DNA and this bias occurred specifically for primers directed to top strand DNA.

Originally, the bisulfite conversion method required an overnight treatment step that is severely damaging to the DNA molecule. Currently, bisulfite conversion lasts two-three hours and is followed by a purification step. There are several commercially available kits for bisulfite treatment. Some studies have compared DNA bisulfite conversion kits that the reader may find helpful. Holmes et al. [20] compared nine different kits from Qiagen (EpiTect Bisulfite, Fast DNA Bisulfite, and Fast FFPE Bisulfite kits); Zymo's (EZ DNA Methylation-Direct, Methylation-Gold, and Methylation-Lightning kits); and Analytik (Jena's innuConvert

Bisulfite Basic, Bisulfite All-In-One, and Bisulfite Body Fluids kits). Dietrich's team evaluated the kits using DNA obtained from fresh tissues, as well as from Formaldehyde Fixed-Paraffin Embedded tissue (FFPE) and large volumes of body fluids. Testing all these kits showed significantly different but comparable results and high performance when applying high concentration of DNA. The differences were observed when applying degraded DNA from FFPE tissues [20]. Though all the kits were found to be adequate, the authors concluded that innuCONVERT Bisulfite All-In-One Kit showed the highest versatility in terms of sample material (DNA, FFPE tissues, cell lines, fresh and frozen tissues, cellular fractions of bronchial aspirates, pleural effusions, ascites, and urine sediment) and had higher DNA yield from formalin-fixed, paraffin-embed tissues without prior extraction [20]. In another study published recently, four bisulfite conversion kits from Diagenode (Premium Bisulfite kit), Qiagen (EpiTect Bisulfite kit), Promega (MethylEdge Bisulfite Conversion System), and Epigentek (BisulFlash DNA Modification kit) were compared. Though some small differences were observed, they were comparable with respect to DNA degradation, conversion efficiency, and conversion specificity. The authors claimed that the best performance was observed with the MethylEdge Bisulfite Conversion System (Promega) followed by the Premium Bisulfite kit (Diagenode) [21]. The final decision of which kit to use is up to a researcher, who should take into account several factors, such as the source of the DNA, the time required for bisulfite conversion, and the cost of the kit.

2.4 Quantifying Bisulfite-Treated DNA

Highly concentrated bisulfite-converted DNA (more than 100 ng/μl) can be crudely measured using the spectrophotometric method. However, this method would be inaccurate with lower concentrations. Methods such as PicoGreen cannot be used to quantify bisulfite-converted DNA since the DNA is single-stranded after bisulfite conversion. The absorption coefficient of bisulfite-treated DNA at 260 nm resembles that of RNA. Therefore, ZymoResearch recommends using a value of 40 μg/mL for OD 260 = 1.0 when determining the concentration of the recovered bisulfite-treated DNA. Qiagen recommends quantifying bisulfite-treated DNA by real-time PCR using methods developed for bisulfite-treated DNA.

To assess the quality and the quantity, the bisulfite-converted DNA can be also run on agarose/EtBr gel. However, with regular DNA running on agarose gel procedure, nothing will be visible in the gel, since DNA after conversion is single-stranded. According to Zymo Research, cooling the gel for 10–15 min in an ice bath will force enough base-pairing to allow intercalation of the ethidium bromide for the DNA to be visible and to allow apparent banding of the DNA. The converted DNA will run as a smear (between 100 and 1500 bp). About 100 ng of bisulfite-converted DNA will be sufficient to be visualized.

**2.5 Primer
and Assay Design**

Assay design is a critical step for successful and accurate DNA methylation quantitative analysis. The aim of this step is to design primers that will allow amplification of the DNA region of interest for each gene and yield a specific PCR product. The pyrosequencing assay involves the design of three primers: forward, reverse (one of which is biotinylated), and sequencing. The Qiagen database offers for purchase more than 84,000 individual assays for the human, mouse, and rat genomes covering more than 80% gene-specific CpG islands. In addition, Qiagen offers predesigned assays for validating methylation arrays, such as Infinium HumanMethylation450 BeadChip array.

A number of commercial and free tools are available for designing pyrosequencing primers. PyroMark Q24 (Qiagen) is commercial software that allows automatic design of forward, reverse, and sequencing primers. Each set of primer is assigned a quality score, reflecting its suitability for pyrosequencing analysis. Primer set is assigned high quality (blue) if no concerns are identified. Though lower quality primer sets should not be excluded, as with additional optimization they may be suitable.

Due to the reduced complexity of the bisulfite-treated DNA, assay design by PyroMark Q24 often leads to failure or a large list of potential errors and complications [22]. Other several free software programs are available for pyrosequencing assay design: MethPrimer [23] (http://www.urogene.org/methprimer/), Bisearch [24] (http://bisearch.enzim.hu/), that uses algorithm proposed by Kämpke et al., for primer design [25], Methyl Primer Express from Applied Biosystems, and CpGWARE primer design software (Chemicon International).

Though the rules for primer design are standard, additional precautions and peculiarities of pyrosequencing reaction should be considered. After identification of the region of interest, PCR primers should be designed according to the following guidelines:

Primer designing rules:

- The recommended amplicon length should be between 150 and 200 bp. However, larger products, up to 350–400 bp, may be successfully sequenced.

- Primer length of about 18–30 bases is required for amplification of bisulfate-converted DNA.

- One of the primers, forward or reverse, should be biotinylated (for immobilization to streptavidin-coated magnetic- or Sepharose in 5′ end). The biotinylated primer should always be complementary to sequencing primer.

- Check primers for potential self-annealing, primer-dimer, or hairpin-loop formation.

- To avoid preferential amplification, primers should not contain any CpGs. If this is unavoidable, then put them in the 5' end of the primer and synthesize them as Y (C/T) in the forward strand and R (G/A) in the reverse stand.

- It is recommended to design primers with at least four cytosines outside of CpG that are converted during bisulfite conversion.

- Primers should be devoid of palindromes (within primers) and complementary sequences between primers to ensure specific amplification.

- Optimal primer melting temperature (Tm) should be between 62 and 65 °C with maximal Tm difference of 10 °C between forward and reverse primers.

- Relatively equal G/C–A/T distribution within the primers.

Primer purification:

- The biotinylated primer needs to be HPLC purified and synthesized at larger scale, whereas non-tagged primers require standard desalting only. HPLC purification of biotinylated primer improves signal strength. HPLC purification minimizes the amount of free biotin, which otherwise will block the binding of biotinylated PCR product to the sepharose or streptavidin beads, that will affect signal intensity during pyrosequencing analysis.

Primer and PCR product storage conditions:

- Biotinylated as well as non-biotinylated primers should be stored at −20 °C. Biotinylated primers are sensitive to thawing/freezing; therefore, aliquoting the primers is recommended and freeze/thaw should not exceed three times.

- Biotinylated PCR products can be stored at 4 °C overnight or at −20 °C for a week.

2.6 PCR of Bisulfite-Treated DNA and Pyrosequencing

After primer and assay design, a DNA fragment of interest should be amplified. PCR is performed with amplification primers, one of which is biotinylated. Accurate PCR amplification is critical for precise evaluation of DNA methylation.

One of the common problems encountered is inaccurate assessment of DNA methylation as a result of PCR bias reflected in preferential amplification of non-methylated DNA over methylated DNA, which can result from a secondary structure formation within the DNA molecule [19].

Since all non-methylated cytosines are converted to uracil, the bisulfite-treated DNA usually is AT-rich and has low GC composition.

Thus, it may be necessary to reduce the annealing temperature accordingly. Therefore, temperature gradient PCR to optimize and find the best annealing temperature condition can significantly enhance the specificity of the product. On the other hand, changing PCR annealing temperature can bias PCR toward amplification of either methylated or unmethylated DNA [26]. Therefore, optimizing annealing temperature alone might not be sufficient. Mixing experiments using varying mixtures of methylated and unmethylated DNA followed by gradient PCR to initially set up, evaluate, and calibrate each new assay is recommended [26]. We found that annealing temperatures between 50 and 60 °C typically work well. Another approach for increasing specificity is using modified PCR protocols such as touchdown PCR (TD-PCR) that uses different annealing temperatures starting with initial annealing temperature that is higher than the optimal Tm and is gradually reduced over subsequent cycles to the Tm temperature or "touchdown temperature." TD-PCR enhances the specificity of the initial primer–template duplex formation and hence the specificity of the final PCR product [27].

We recommend the use of HotStar Taq DNA polymerase (Table 1) to amplify specific bisulfate-converted sequences, which compared to regular Taq polymerase diminish spurious DNA amplification, primer-dimers, and background. For DNA regions that have a high degree of secondary structure or high GC-content, using Q-Solution (Qiagen), which changes DNA melting behavior, can improve PCR reaction. The need for this step can be tested for each primer/template setup, by running parallel PCR reactions with and without Q-Solution under the same cycling conditions and then subsequently visualizing all products on agarose gels.

It is highly recommended to use a negative control for the detection of DNA contamination in the reaction mixture components or the water. It is also recommended to include

Table 1
PCR reaction setup using HotStar Taq DNA polymerase

Component	Volume/reaction (μl)	Concentration per reaction
Bisulfite-treated DNA (DNA input before conversion-50 ng/μl)	1	50 ng
10× PCR buffer	5	1× (contains 15 mM MgCl$_2$)
dNTP mix (10 mM each)	1	200 μM of each dNTP
Primer forward (10 μM)	1	0.5 μM
Primer reverse (10 μM)	1	0.5 μM
HotStar Taq DNA polymerase (5U/μl)	0.25	1.25 U/reaction
PCR grade H$_2$O	—	up to 50 μl

positive controls: unmethylated, fully methylated, and hemi-methylated DNA (by mixing in equal proportion fully and unmethylated DNA). Unmethylated and fully methylated DNA are commercially available. Fully methylated DNA can be also enzymatically modified in vitro with CpG Methylase (M.SssI), whereas whole genome amplification (WGA) enables amplification of an entire genome in the absence of methylation and produces unmethylated DNA.

The following thermocycler program is used with HotStar Taq DNA polymerase: 95 °C for 15 min that enable initial heat activation of polymerase, followed by 45–50 cycles of 94 °C for 1 min, varying annealing temperature for 45 s and 72 °C extension for 1 min. Final extension at 72 °C for 10 min.

After completing the PCR reaction, run the PCR product on 1.5 % agarose gel. It is critical to have a strong single band without nonspecific products and primer-dimers, as this can affect sequencing results.

The obtained biotinylated PCR product serves as a substrate for the subsequent pyrosequencing reaction. We carry out Pyrosequencing with PyroMark Gold reagents (Qiagen) on a PyroMark Q24 or Q96md pyrosequencer (Qiagen), following the manufacturer's recommendations. Pyrosequencing requires a single stranded sequencing template. Amplification of DNA fragment of interest with one of the biotinylated primers is followed by capturing amplified template with streptavidin beads and the non-biotinylated strand is removed following denaturing with NaOH. After strand elution and subsequent washings to remove all other reaction components, the sequencing primer is added and annealed to the pure single stranded DNA template.

If sequencing is not complete, i.e., sequence primer location does not allow covering all CpGs of interest then serial pyrosequencing can be used, where multiple sequencing primers can be designed. In this case, the PCR template can be reused after initial sequencing and sequenced with several sequencing primers without the need to perform additional PCR amplifications. In addition to saving labor time and accelerating the workflow, this method has other obvious advantages, such as reduction of the required amount of enzyme and substrates; the cartridge can be reused without washing between the runs and 60 μL of each reagent can be subtracted from the required volumes. It is possible to use three-four sequencing primers, which may cover the whole sequencing of the entire amplified template [28].

2.7 Quantitative Methylated DNA Immunoprecipitation (qMeDIP)

Methylated DNA immunoprecipitation is a method based on enrichment used to delineate the methylation status of DNA regions, first introduced in 2005 by Weber et al., [29]. MeDIP utilizes an anti-5mC antibody and captures 250–1000 bp fragments of DNA. Downstream application of MeDIP includes next generation sequencing and microarray as described in Chap. 1 or real-time quantitative PCR (qPCR). QMeDIP combines MeDIP and traditional qPCR, allowing one to determine the relative enrichment of DNA methylation in fragments assessed for particular loci. In comparison to MeDIP-seq or MeDIP-ChIP as described in Chapter #1, qMeDIP is relatively quick and cost effective. However, this technique is only useful for known target genes, as specific primer sets must be designed to interrogate these genes. Further, immunoprecipitated material is limited, thus creating a bottleneck for the number of target loci that may be examined. In contrast to bisulfite conversion-based methods that provide a single CpG resolution, MeDIP assesses the methylation status within the DNA fragments and thus provides only regional information. As such, MeDIP cannot discern the number of CpGs within a region that are methylated. Detailed comparisons between MeDIP and sodium bisulfite conversion can be found in Chap. 1. The extraction of high quality genomic DNA is a critical first step required for all downstream applications when assessing the methylome, particularly for MeDIP as the quality of genomic DNA may affect antibody binding and thus the downstream steps and quality and reliability of the data generated (DNA extraction and concentration measurements are discussed in the "Pyrosequencing" section 2.2).

A minimum of 2 μg of starting genomic DNA is recommended to proceed with qMeDIP. Following assessment of quality and quantity, genomic DNA shearing is required. The Bioruptor® (Diagenode) is recommended to reduce fragment size to a range between 250 and 1000 bp; a concentration of 0.01 μg/μl genomic DNA is recommended. Fragment size should be confirmed with gel electrophoresis. Following genomic DNA shearing, fragmented DNA is diluted with TE (10 mM Tris–HCl pH 7.5, 1 mM EDTA, ~7×) and boiled at 95 °C for 10 min to heat-denature into single-stranded DNA. The sample should be cooled immediately to avoid re-annealing of strands. An aliquot is then removed and frozen for later use, representing the "input" (containing methylated and nonmethylated fragments). The remaining sample is precleared and incubated with 5-methyl-cytosine (5mC) antibody and incubated overnight. One potential bias, as with any protocols that require the use of antibody, is specificity. The most commonly used antibody is a mouse monocolonal anti-5mC from Eurogenetec. The affinity of this anti-5mC toward 5mC in comparison to hydroxymethylation (5hmC) has been validated [30]. Postincubation, Protein G magnetic beads are added and the reaction mix is incubated on a rotator for 2 h at 4 °C. The single-stranded DNA bound to 5mC antibody will be captured by the magnetic beads and later subsequently incubated with digestion buffer (50 mM Tris–HCl pH 8; 10 mM EDTA, 0.5% SDS and

20–40 μg Proteinase K) to release the "bound" fraction. Finally, DNA purification of all fractions is required and can be performed by phenol–chloroform or column-based purification methods.

2.8 Primer Design

Primer design for qMeDIP follows the same basic principles as regular primer design for qPCR. Briefly, primers should be designed so that amplicon size is <200 bp, melting temperature is around 60 °C, the GC content is around 50–60%, and the two primers should have low self-complementarity to reduce the possibility of primer-dimer formation [31]. In addition, primers should be ideally designed so that there are no CpG sites in the actual primer. Numerous free online software is available to aid in primer design including: Primer3 (http://bioinfo.ut.ee/primer3-0.4.0/) and AutoPrime (http://www.autoprime.de/AutoPrimeWeb) [32]. Once the reverse and forward primers are designed, it is recommended to check the product specificity by running a primer BLAST on NCBI (http://www.ncbi.nlm.nih.gov/tools/primer-blast/) or the USCS Genome Browser.

2.9 Analysis

To assess the efficacy of the immunoprecipitation, qPCR, comparing the bound fraction to input for specific loci is often performed using controls. The promoter of imprinted genes, such as *H19*, is commonly used as a "positive" control normalized to housekeeping genes, such as *GAPDH*, which have minimal or no methylation [33]. Additional control sequences that are highly methylated include *Xist* and *LAP*, unmethylated include *Actb* and *Aprt* or regions that lack CpG sites (*CSa* and *CSb*) [29]. Alternatively, spiking samples with unmethylated and methylated plasmids (6 pg of each) prior to sonication is advisable. Following immunoprecipitation, qPCR can be performed on suing primers specific to the methylated and unmethylated plasmids to validate input and bound fractions [34]. Additional spike-in approaches are available and primer sequences have been developed [35]. Ideally, the input Ct should not exceed 30. Enrichment (E) can be calculated as follows; $E = (B_{target}/I_{target})/(B_{negative\ control}/I_{negative\ control})$ where "target" is the methylated region of interest and "negative control" is an unmethylated DNA region.

2.10 High Resolution Melting for Data Validation of Genome-Wide DNA Methylation Studies

High resolution melting is a post-PCR technique that measures changes in fluorescence levels as a function of double-strand dissociation caused by an increasing melting gradient. The use of an in-tube assay that combines real-time PCR and subsequent high resolution melting (HRM) was first introduced in 1997 [36] and was later reported for methylation analysis in 2001 [2]. An improvement of the technique, methylation-sensitive HRM (MS-HRM), has later been introduced, which provides increased sensitivity for the detection of methylation and makes compensation for possible PCR bias [37, 38].

HRM is based on double-strand melting and contemporary fluorescent measurements that are collected from the release of an intercalating double-stranded DNA-specific dye and visualized as a melting profile. DNA strands with different base compositions have different melting profiles. After sodium bisulfite treatment of a DNA sequence, unmethylated cytosines are converted to uracils while methylated cytosines remain unchanged and hence, melting profiles will reflect the methylation status of the DNA sequence.

2.11   Protocol

The protocol for MS-HRM is outlined in the following passages and the principles behind the method are illustrated in Fig. 1. Purified genomic DNA is treated with sodium bisulfite (DNA extraction and concentration measurements followed by bisulfite conversion are discussed in the Pyrosequencing section) and used as input for PCR. Primers are designed to anneal to the sodium bisulfate-treated DNA. The base composition of the amplified sequence between the primers will determine the melting profile visualized in the melting phase.

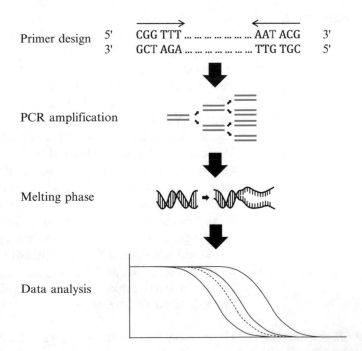

Fig. 1 Schematic workflow for MS-HRM. Specific primers for MS-HRM are designed to only one of the bisulfate-treated DNA sequences. Thymines marked in red correspond to unmethylated cytosines. When optimal instrumentation is available, the PCR amplification and the melting phase are performed as an integrated process. Double-strand disassociation of the melting phase is measured as a drop of fluorescence, which is illustrated in the subsequent data analysis. The methylation level of a DNA sample of unknown level (*dotted line*) is estimated by comparison of the melting profiles derived from standards of known methylation level (*solid lines*)

2.12 Primer Design

A critical step in MS-HRM is primer design. Primers are designed to only one of the strands, since the strands are no longer complementary after sodium bisulfite treatment. Bias toward preferred amplification of the unmethylated template is a well-known problem in PCR-based methods for analyzing DNA methylation [19]. This bias can be compensated by designing primers that are fully complementary to the methylated template with a single or two CpG sites as close to the 5'-end as possible and by adjusting the annealing temperature in a subsequent optimization process [37, 38]. When a CpG site is included in a primer it reduces the affinity for binding to the unmethylated template by causing a mismatch. If the annealing temperature is increased, the affinity for the unmethylated template will be further reduced. In addition to reducing PCR bias, the adjustment of annealing temperature increases the sensitivity of the assay and enables identification of methylation in an unmethylated background down to 0.1% [39]. Unusual PCR bias toward preferred amplification of the methylated template can occur for regions of interest where high methylation levels are expected. In MS-HRM analysis of imprinted genes, PCR bias toward the methylated template may appear [40]. Hence, it has a negative impact to favor annealing to the methylated template and it should be considered to design primers fully complementary to the unmethylated template instead.

In addition to the specific recommendations for MS-HRM, the following rules for primer design should be applied:

- Melting temperature of the primers should be matched within 1–2 °C.

- Non-CpG cytosines should be included in 3'-end of primers to avoid amplification of nonconverted DNA.

- Primers should be above 20 bp in length. Sodium bisulfite treatment reduces complexity of the DNA and longer primers are needed for specificity compared to PCR of non-bisulfate-treated template.

- Amplicon size should not exceed 100 bp to reduce complexity of the melting profile.

- General recommendations on how to avoid formation of primer-dimer and secondary structure should be followed.

MS-HRM can theoretically detect methylation at a single CpG site, but a better resolution is achieved when additional CpG sites are included. Wojdacz et al. [41] recommend 6-8 CpG sites between the primers to avoid unambiguous melting profiles. Interpretation of the data is impeded if more melting domains appear which is often caused if the amplicons are too large or if too many CpG sites are included. Hence, the designing of an optimal assay will often balance between obtaining the maximal resolution between the melting profiles while maintaining a simple melting profile.

Table 2
An overview of reagents required for MS-HRM

Component	Concentration per reaction
Forward primer	200–300 nM
Reverse primer	200–300 nM
Bisulfite-converted DNA template	10–20 ng
$MgCl_2$	2–4 mM
dsDNA intercalating Dye	2–4 μM
Hot-Start Taq DNA polymerase	0.5 U
dNTPs	0.2 mM
PCR buffer	1×
PCR grade H_2O	up to 20 μl

2.13 **Input and Setup**   Table 2 shows an overview of reagents required for MS-HRM. A Hot-Start polymerase is preferred as it reduces the possibility of nonspecific products and primer-dimer formation. It is important to choose a dye that does not inhibit the PCR reaction in saturating concentrations. The use of a dye in a saturating concentration prevents redistribution of the dyes to more stable duplexes during the melting phase [42]. Some of the most often used dyes applicable for MS-HRM are LCGREEN (BioFire Defense, USA) EvaGreen (Biotium, USA), SYTO9 (Life Technologies, USA), and ResoLight (Roche Applied Science, Germany), which can be all used in saturating concentrations without inhibiting the PCR reactions [43, 44].

A standard dilution series of fully methylated template that is mixed with unmethylated template have to be included in every experimental run. The standard dilution series of known methylation level is used to estimate the methylation level of a sample in a semiquantitative manner. The level of the sample is estimated by comparison with the melting profiles of the standards. A standard containing equal amounts of unmethylated and methylated templates should always be included to estimate the extent of PCR bias.

For each experiment, a negative control without template should be included to control for contamination. In addition, a control containing unmodified genomic DNA as a template can be included to ensure that the amplified DNA originate from sodium bisulfite-treated DNA. No amplification should be observed in any of the above-mentioned controls. The amplification of unmodified genomic DNA can be prevented by including non-CpG cytosines in the 3′ end of the primer design [41]. The real-time detection of the PCR amplification serves as a control for equal amounts of DNA before the melting phase. The number of PCR cycles can be increased to ensure that all reactions have reached the plateau phase before melting.

A typical PCR protocol for MS-HRM is as follows: 10 min of preheating at 95 °C followed by 50 repeated cycles of: 10 s at 95 °C, 15 s at the annealing temperature optimized for the assay, and 10 s at 72 °C. The annealing temperature can be changed to reduce PCR bias, to increase sensitivity, or to obtain a better resolution for a desired temperature. We suggest using an annealing temperature about 5 °C below the melting temperature for the initial PCR. The HRM phase is initiated with a 1 min melting phase at 95 °C followed by cool down to 65 °C to allow hybridization. Subsequently, the double-stranded DNA is melted by a 0.2 °C/s temperature increasing ramp until the temperature reaches 95 °C.

It is recommended to combine the two processes, real-time PCR and MS-HRM, in a single instrument containing a real-time thermocycler and optics capable of collecting fluorescent data points. It minimizes the risk of contamination, is the simplest way of performing the assay, and enables the real-time data to serve as a control for equal amounts of DNA before the melting phase. The Lightcycler 480 (Roche), Rotor-Gene Q (Qiagen) earlier available as Rotor-Gene 6000 (Corbett Life Science), 7500 Fast Real-Time PCR system (Applied Biosystems), and 7900HT Fast Real-Time PCR System (Applied Biosystems) are all suitable for this technique.

2.14 Data Analysis

Post-PCR raw data are interpreted when plotted as normalized fluorescence against temperature or as the negative first derivative against temperature. Each way of visualizing the data is shown in Fig. 2.

The specific melting temperature for a sample is determined as the temperature corresponding to the sharpest drop of fluorescence for the normalized melting curve or as the peak of the profile for the negative first derivative. After sodium bisulfite treatment, a sample of originally high methylation level will have a higher melting temperature than one of unmethylated origin due to a higher content of remaining cytosines in the methylated sample. The methylation level of an unknown sample is then estimated in a semiquantitative way by comparison of the specific melting profile with melting profiles derived from standard series of DNA with known methylation level.

An advantage of MS-HRM is the ability to detect heterogeneous methylation [2]. In contrast to the analysis of homogenous methylation, the analysis of heterogeneous methylation by MS-HRM is qualitative [45]. The template of heterogeneous methylated origin will be visualized as a broad melting profile

a)   b)

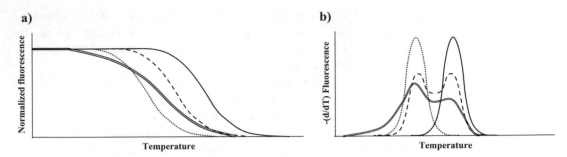

Fig. 2 MS-HRM data visualized as either (**a**) normalized fluorescence against temperature or (**b**) the negative derivative against temperature. The *dotted line* represents an unmethylated template. The intact line represents a fully methylated template. The *dashed line* represents a template of equal amounts of methylated and unmethylated origin. The two-lined melting profile represents a sample of heterogeneous methylated origin

where melting begins before the unmethylated standard due to the formation of heteroduplexes with insufficient base pairing which is illustrated in Fig. 2. If quantification of heterogeneous methylation is desired for a larger number of regions of interest, MS-HRM can be used as a powerful screening tool to detect complex methylation patterns in a single sample. By using biotinylated primers for MS-HRM, the PCR product can subsequently be used as input for bisulfite pyrosequencing which will provide quantitative information about heterogeneous methylation [46].

PCR bias in the assay is detected by analyzing standard dilutions of equal amounts of methylated and unmethylated templates. Preferred amplification of one of the templates can be detected if the melt peak analysis does not show equal heights of the peaks corresponding to each template. An increase of the annealing temperature will shift the primer affinity toward the methylated template and increase the sensitivity of the assay [41].

2.15 Conclusion for MS-HRM

MS-HRM is a simple and cost-efficient way to validate genome-wide methylation data. After the optimization of the assay, the technique provides a robust tool to analyze a large number of samples during a short time with low associated expenses and demands for equipment. However, MS-HRM does not provide information about methylation at a single-site resolution. In that case, we recommend other techniques such as bisulfite sequencing [18] or pyrosequencing [47]. MS-HRM provides significant agreement of quantification and qualification of DNA methylation with other highly recognized techniques like pyrosequencing and bisulfite sequencing [39, 48, 49]. Therefore, in validation studies where semiquantitative methylation values are sufficient and high-throughput and cost-effectiveness are desired, MS-HRM should be the method of choice.

Acknowledgments

D.C. is supported by fellowship from the Israel Cancer Research Foundation. S.P. is supported by the Mats Sundin Fellowship in Developmental Health.

References

1. Ronaghi M et al (1998) PCR-introduced loop structure as primer in DNA sequencing. Biotechniques 25(5):876, -8, 880-2, 884

2. Worm J, Aggerholm A, Guldberg P (2001) In-tube DNA methylation profiling by fluorescence melting curve analysis. Clin Chem 47(7):1183–1189

3. Xiong Z, Laird PW (1997) COBRA: a sensitive and quantitative DNA methylation assay. Nucleic Acids Res 25(12):2532–2534

4. Ronaghi M, Uhlen M, Nyren P (1998) A sequencing method based on real-time pyrophosphate. Science 281(5375):363, 365

5. Langaee T, Ronaghi M (2005) Genetic variation analyses by Pyrosequencing. Mutat Res 573(1-2):96–102

6. Ogino S et al (2005) Sensitive sequencing method for KRAS mutation detection by Pyrosequencing. J Mol Diagn 7(3):413–421

7. Ronaghi M (2001) Pyrosequencing sheds light on DNA sequencing. Genome Res 11(1):3–11

8. Sanger F, Coulson AR (1975) A rapid method for determining sequences in DNA by primed synthesis with DNA polymerase. J Mol Biol 94(3):441–448

9. Petropoulos S, Matthews SG, Szyf M (2014) Adult glucocorticoid exposure leads to transcriptional and DNA methylation changes in nuclear steroid receptors in the hippocampus and kidney of mouse male offspring. Biol Reprod 90(2):43

10. Kirby KS (1956) A new method for the isolation of ribonucleic acids from mammalian tissues. Biochem J 64(3):405–408

11. Ebeling W et al (1974) Proteinase K from Tritirachium album Limber. Eur J Biochem 47(1):91–97

12. Manchester KL (1996) Use of UV methods for measurement of protein and nucleic acid concentrations. Biotechniques 20(6):968–970

13. Glasel JA (1995) Validity of nucleic acid purities monitored by 260nm/280nm absorbance ratios. Biotechniques 18(1):62–63

14. Huberman JA (1995) Importance of measuring nucleic acid absorbance at 240 nm as well as at 260 and 280 nm. Biotechniques 18(4):636

15. Manchester KL (1995) Value of A260/A280 ratios for measurement of purity of nucleic acids. Biotechniques 19(2):208–210

16. Hayatsu H et al (1970) Reaction of sodium bisulfite with uracil, cytosine, and their derivatives. Biochemistry 9(14):2858–2865

17. Robert Shapiro RES, Welcher M (1970) Reactions of uracil and cytosine derivatives with sodium bisulfite. J Am Chem Soc 92(2):422–424

18. Frommer M et al (1992) A genomic sequencing protocol that yields a positive display of 5-methylcytosine residues in individual DNA strands. Proc Natl Acad Sci U S A 89(5):1827–1831

19. Warnecke PM et al (1997) Detection and measurement of PCR bias in quantitative methylation analysis of bisulphite-treated DNA. Nucleic Acids Res 25(21):4422–4426

20. Holmes EE et al (2014) Performance evaluation of kits for bisulfite-conversion of DNA from tissues, cell lines, FFPE tissues, aspirates, lavages, effusions, plasma, serum, and urine. PLoS One 9(4):e93933

21. Leontiou CA et al (2015) Bisulfite conversion of DNA: performance comparison of different kits and methylation quantitation of epigenetic biomarkers that have the potential to be used in non-invasive prenatal testing. PLoS One 10(8):e0135058

22. Tost J, Gut IG (2007) DNA methylation analysis by pyrosequencing. Nat Protoc 2(9):2265–2275

23. Li LC, Dahiya R (2002) MethPrimer: designing primers for methylation PCRs. Bioinformatics 18(11):1427–1431

24. Aranyi T et al (2006) The BiSearch web server. BMC Bioinformatics 7:431

25. Kampke T, Kieninger M, Mecklenburg M (2001) Efficient primer design algorithms. Bioinformatics 17(3):214–225

26. Shen L, et al. (2007) Optimizing annealing temperature overcomes bias in bisulfite PCR methylation analysis. Biotechniques 42(1): 48, 50, 52 passim

27. Korbie DJ, Mattick JS (2008) Touchdown PCR for increased specificity and sensitivity in PCR amplification. Nat Protoc 3(9):1452–1456

28. Tost J, El abdalaoui H, Gut IG (2006) Serial pyrosequencing for quantitative DNA methylation analysis. Biotechniques 40(6): 721–722, 724, 726

29. Weber M et al (2005) Chromosome-wide and promoter-specific analyses identify sites of differential DNA methylation in normal and transformed human cells. Nat Genet 37(8): 853–862

30. Jin SG, Kadam S, Pfeifer GP (2010) Examination of the specificity of DNA methylation profiling techniques towards 5-methylcytosine and 5-hydroxymethylcytosine. Nucleic Acids Res 38(11):e125

31. Bustin SA et al (2009) The MIQE guidelines: minimum information for publication of quantitative real-time PCR experiments. Clin Chem 55(4):611–622

32. Wrobel G, Kokocinski F, Lichter P (2004) AutoPrime: selecting primers for expressed sequences. Genome Biol 5(5):P11

33. Petropoulos S et al (2015) Gestational diabetes alters offspring DNA methylation profiles in human and rat: identification of key pathways involved in endocrine system disorders, insulin signaling, diabetes signaling, and ILK signaling. Endocrinology 156(6):2222–2238

34. Labonte B et al (2012) Genome-wide epigenetic regulation by early-life trauma. Arch Gen Psychiatry 69(7):722–731

35. Lisanti S, von Zglinicki T, Mathers JC (2012) Standardization and quality controls for the methylated DNA immunoprecipitation technique. Epigenetics 7(6):615–625

36. Wittwer CT et al (1997) The LightCycler: a microvolume multisample fluorimeter with rapid temperature control. Biotechniques 22(1):176–181

37. Wojdacz TK, Dobrovic A (2007) Methylation-sensitive high resolution melting (MS-HRM): a new approach for sensitive and high-throughput assessment of methylation. Nucleic Acids Res 35(6), e41

38. Wojdacz TK, Hansen LL (2006) Reversal of PCR bias for improved sensitivity of the DNA methylation melting curve assay. Biotechniques 41(3):274, 276, 278

39. Wojdacz TK et al (2010) Limitations and advantages of MS-HRM and bisulfite sequencing for single locus methylation studies. Expert Rev Mol Diagn 10(5):575–580

40. Rubatino FV et al (2015) Manipulation of primer affinity improves high-resolution melting accuracy for imprinted genes. Genet Mol Res 14(3):7864–7872

41. Wojdacz TK, Dobrovic A, Hansen LL (2008) Methylation-sensitive high-resolution melting. Nat Protoc 3(12):1903–1908

42. Wittwer CT et al (2003) High-resolution genotyping by amplicon melting analysis using LCGreen. Clin Chem 49(6 Pt 1):853–860

43. Monis PT, Giglio S, Saint CP (2005) Comparison of SYTO9 and SYBR Green I for real-time polymerase chain reaction and investigation of the effect of dye concentration on amplification and DNA melting curve analysis. Anal Biochem 340(1):24–34

44. Radvanszky J et al (2015) Comparison of different DNA binding fluorescent dyes for applications of high-resolution melting analysis. Clin Biochem 48(9):609–616

45. Candiloro IL et al (2008) Rapid analysis of heterogeneously methylated DNA using digital methylation-sensitive high resolution melting: application to the CDKN2B (p15) gene. Epigenetics Chromatin 1(1):7

46. Candiloro IL, Mikeska T, Dobrovic A (2011) Assessing combined methylation-sensitive high resolution melting and pyrosequencing for the analysis of heterogeneous DNA methylation. Epigenetics 6(4):500–507

47. Ronaghi M et al (1996) Real-time DNA sequencing using detection of pyrophosphate release. Anal Biochem 242(1):84–89

48. Amornpisutt R, Sriraksa R, Limpaiboon T (2012) Validation of methylation-sensitive high resolution melting for the detection of DNA methylation in cholangiocarcinoma. Clin Biochem 45(13–14):1092–1094

49. Migheli F et al (2013) Comparison study of MS-HRM and pyrosequencing techniques for quantification of APC and CDKN2A gene methylation. PLoS One 8(1):e52501

Chapter 4

Analyzing Targeted Nucleosome Position and Occupancy in Cancer, Obesity, and Diabetes

Prasad P. Devarshi and Tara M. Henagan

Abstract

Chromatin structure plays an integral role in regulation of gene transcription. Studying nucleosome position and occupancy at key regulatory regions within DNA is important to understanding the potential epigenetic mechanisms of gene regulation during various environmental exposures and diseased states. Targeted nucleosome mapping is a convenient method to map nucleosome positions at a specific genomic locus. In this method, mononucleosomal DNA is isolated using micrococcal nuclease. This is followed by qPCR, which uses the mononucleosomal DNA, or the DNA bound by the nucleosome, as the template and overlapping primers that span the target region of genome. qPCR products are analyzed by gel electrophoresis and densitometry to yield a map of nucleosomes along specific, targeted genomic loci.

Key words Nucleosome, Epigenetics, Scanning PCR, Cancer, Obesity, Type 2 diabetes

1 Introduction

1.1 Role of Epigenetics and Chromatic Structure in Cancer, Obesity, and Diabetes

Epigenetics is the study of heritable changes in gene expression that occur independent of DNA sequence modifications. Epigenetic mechanisms include DNA methylation, posttranslational histone modifications, and microRNAs [1–3]. Each epigenetic modification plays an intricate role in making up the epigenetic code and determining conformation of the DNA structure and compaction into chromatin [4]. Epigenetic modifications determine the chromatin structure partially through altering the basic subunit of DNA, the nucleosome. Histone methylation, acetylation, sumolyation, phosphorylation, and ubiquitination, as well as DNA methylation, have the potential to alter nucleosome positioning and occupancy [5–9]. The nucleosome positioning and occupancy play significant roles in regulation of gene expression [10]. Nucleosomes can block access of transcription factors and the transcription machinery to their binding sites on the DNA. For example, binding of the TATA-binding protein to the DNA is inhibited if a nucleosome is present at the locus of the TATA box,

Barbara Stefanska and David J. MacEwan (eds.), *Epigenetics and Gene Expression in Cancer, Inflammatory and Immune Diseases*, Methods in Pharmacology and Toxicology, DOI 10.1007/978-1-4939-6743-8_4, © Springer Science+Business Media LLC 2017

further inhibiting recruitment of RNA polymerase II [11]. Furthermore, changes in nucleosomal positioning at the promoter region can affect gene transcription [12, 13]. Nucleosome occupancy is generally decreased upstream of transcriptionally active genes and increased upstream of repressed genes [14, 15]. If a nucleosome is positioned at the -1 position, meaning it is the first nucleosome upstream of the transcriptional start site, it can prevent the binding of regulatory proteins to the transcription controller, the *cis*-regulatory element [16]. Conversely, nucleosomes may promote gene expression by mediating protein–protein interactions that are necessary for transcription initiation [17]. Nucleosomes may also reciprocally regulate the epigenetic code [18]. The positioning of nucleosomes is regulated by histone affinities to DNA sequences [19] and the activity of ATP-dependent remodeling complexes [20] and various other proteins [21, 22], all of which are fundamentally dependent on the epigenetic modifications at a specific locus.

Epigenetic modifications and nucleosome positioning and occupancy play a significant role in disease onset and progression, as indicated in cancer, obesity and type 2 diabetes. For example, mutL homolog 1 (MLH1), an essential gene in the DNA mismatch repair system, is silenced in cancer cells due to presence of three nucleosomes in the promoter region that are absent in non-cancer cells [23]. In acute promyelocytic leukemia, the leukemogenic protein promyelocytic leukemia/retinoic acid receptor alpha, recruits nucleosome remodeling and deacetylase corepressor complex (NuRD), which epigenetically silences the tumor-suppressor gene, retinoic acid receptor beta 2 (RARβ2) via chromatin remodeling [24]; and AT-rich interactive domain-containing protein 1A (ARID1A), a component of the SWI/SNF chromatin-remodeling complex, is mutated in ovarian clear cell carcinoma cells, suggesting that abnormal chromatin remodeling is involved in the pathogenesis of this cancer [25]. Additionally, alterations in DNA methylation and histone acetylation have been noted in obesity and type 2 diabetes, disease states highly induced by environmental factors such as nutrition and exercise [26–28]. In our own work, we have observed that in overweight and obese individuals, skeletal muscle -1 nucleosome positioning with the gene peroxisome proliferator alpha receptor gamma coactivator 1 alpha (*PGC1α*) is associated with cardiovascular disease risk [29]. We and others have also observed that high fat diets, leading to obesity and type 2 diabetes, alters whole genome nucleosome maps and epigenomes, resulting in aberrant gene expression, phenotypes and physiologies [30–32]. Specifically, high fat diet-induced -1 nucleosome positioning in skeletal muscle nuclear-encoded mitochondrial genes, such as *PGC1α*, seems to play a major role in determining in mitochondrial adaptations that contribute to obesity and type 2 diabetes [30].

Given the role of epigenetics, including nucleosome positioning and occupancy, in disease onset and progression, here we aim to describe a detailed methodology to determine nucleosome position and occupancy using scanning qPCR. Nucleosome scanning assay involves the isolation of mononucleosomal DNA using micrococcal nuclease (MNase) followed by qPCR to detect nucleosome occupancy and positioning. It is a relatively convenient and rapid procedure. It can provide high-resolution nucleosome maps at targeted genomic loci, and thus can be used to study individual promoters or other genomic loci in detail. It is a tool which can help us gain new insights into complex physiological processes. Analyzing nucleosome maps can help us understand which genomic loci are targeted for epigenetic regulation in various diseases and the potential epigenetic mechanisms involved. Qualification and quantification of nucleosome positioning and occupancy may allow us to determine whether specific interventions, such as alterations in diet or exercise, may reverse aberrant nucleosome positioning, leading to more beneficial phenotypes and physiologies, in various diseases.

2 Materials

2.1 Equipment

Pipettes.

Thermocycler (conventional and real time).

Analytical balance.

Cooling tabletop centrifuge.

Gel imager.

Agarose gel cast.

ImageJ software.

Mechanical homogenizer.

4 °C refrigerator.

−20°C and −80 °C freezers.

NanoDrop spectrophotometer.

2.2 General Materials for All Applications

Pipette Tips.

1.5 mL tubes.

Ice buckets.

Ice.

Spatulas.

Weigh boats.

diH$_2$O.

Nuclease-free water.

2.3 **Materials**	Flash frozen tissue samples.
2.3.1 *Mononucleosomal DNA Isolation and Purification*	Liquid nitrogen in small dewar.

Mortar and pestle.

Tin foil cut into squares that fit in the mortar and cover the sides and bottom.

1 mL Dounce homogenizer.

Micrococcal nuclease (MNase; Roche, Basel, Switzerland) at 20 U.

Proteinase K, prepared at 0.1 mg/mL (Qiagen, Valencia, CA).

Heat block at 37 °C.

Heat block at 55 °C.

Agarose.

EtBR.

2.3.2 Scanning qPCR

0.5 mL tubes.

Adhesive films.

Mononucleosomal DNA samples.

Genomic DNA samples.

Primer pairs spanning region of interest.

PCR Master Mix.

2.4 **Buffers**

2.4.1 Sucrose Buffer (100 mL).

0.25 M sucrose.

10 mM Tris–acetate.

1 mM EDTA.

1 mM DTT.

1 mM sodium orthovanadate.

1×, EDTA-free protease inhibitor cocktail tablet (Roche 11873580001).

2.4.2 Digestion Buffer (50 mL)

0.25 M sucrose buffer.

4 mM $MgCl_2$.

1 mM $CaCl_2$.

2.4.3 Lysis Buffer (50 mL)

50 mM Tris–acetate pH 8.1

10 mM EDTA.

1% SDS.

1×, EDTA-free protease inhibitor cocktail tablet (Roche 11873580001).

2.4.4 0.2 M EDTA (1 mL)

0.0074 g EDTA in 1 mL $ddiH_2O$.

Use immediately or store at −20 °C.

3   Methods

3.1 Sucrose Buffer Preparation

To make the sucrose buffer, several stock components are needed, including: 200 mM sodium orthovanadate, 500 mM DTT, 100 mM EDTA and 1 M Tris–acetate. First make a 200 mM sodium orthovanadate solution by dissolving 1.839 g sodium orthovanadate into 50 mL ddiH$_2$O. Adjust the pH to 10, and boil the yellow solution until it turns clear. Adjust pH to 10 again. Aliquot and store at -80C. Make a 500 mM stock of DTT by dissolving 0.77 g powder in 10 mL ddiH$_2$O, aliquot and store at -80C. Make a 100 mM EDTA stock by dissolving 0.292 g EDTA in 10 mL ddiH$_2$O. Store at room temperature. Make 1 M stock solution of Tris–acetate, pH 8.1 by dissolving 12.114 g Tris in 10 mL ddiH$_2$O and pH to 8.1 with acetate. Store at room temperature or 4°C to prevent growth. Once all stock components are ready, the 0.25 sucrose solution can be made by first dissolving 8.56 g of sucrose into 100 mL ddiH$_2$O, giving 0.25 M sucrose. Take 70 mL of the sucrose solution and add 1 mL of 1 M stock solution of Tris–acetate pH 8.1 to give a final 10 mM concentration of Tris–acetate. Add 1 mL of 100 mM stock EDTA (1 mM final) to the buffer. Add 200uL of 500 mM DTT (1 mM final) to the buffer. Add 500 µL of 200 mM sodium orthovanadate (1 mM final) to the buffer. Bring the final volume up to 100 mL with remaining 0.25 M sucrose solution. Remove 50 mL of the sucrose buffer and dissolve in 1 protease inhibitor tablet (1×, complete EDTA-free). Use the sucrose buffer immediately or store at −20 °C for future use. Keep the remaining 50 mL of sucrose buffer (without protease inhibitors) to use for the digestion buffer outlined below.

3.2 Digestion Buffer Preparation

To make the digestion buffer, make the 0.25 M sucrose buffer as outlined above in the sucrose buffer section or use remaining 50 mL of 0.25 M sucrose buffer (without protease inhibitors). Add MgCl$_2$ to a final concentration of 4 mM (0.019 g in 50 mL sucrose buffer) and CaCl$_2$ to a final concentration of 1 mM (0.006 g in 50 mL sucrose buffer) into the 50 mL of 0.25 M sucrose. Use the digestion buffer immediately or store at −20 °C.

3.3 Lysis Buffer Preparation

To make the lysis buffer, first make a stock of 50 mM Tris–acetate, pH 8.1 by dissolving 0.305 g Tris in 100 mL ddiH$_2$O and pH to 8.1 with acetate. Add EDTA to a final concentration of 10 mM (0.145 g in 50 mL Tris–acetate buffer) and SDS to a final concentration of 1 % (0.5 mL in 50 mL Tris–acetate). Bring the solution up to 50 mL with ddiH$_2$O. Add 1 protease inhibitor tablet (1×, complete EDTA-free) to the solution. Use the lysis buffer immediately or store at 4 °C.

3.4 Mono-nucleosomal DNA Isolation and Purification

3.4.1 Frozen Tissue Sample Preparation

All steps for DNA isolation should be performed on ice as necessary. To prepare for the isolation, first take out 2 mL Dounce homogenizers and 1.5 mL tubes and place on ice to cool. Place 0.25 M sucrose buffer on ice. Care should be taken to prevent DNA degradation in tissue samples, by keeping samples cool throughout the procedure. Previously snap-frozen tissues are used in this protocol for native DNA isolation. To begin DNA isolation, remove tissue samples from −80 °C freezer and keep frozen in liquid nitrogen or take samples out of the freezer one at a time to process. In our laboratory, we have found that by placing precut squares of aluminum foil inside a mortar, such that the foil covers the sides and bottom of the mortar, we are able to keep samples cool and also create a vehicle for easy transport of crushed tissue samples into 1.5 mL tubes. Thus, we next place a square of aluminum foil in a mortar, making sure to cover the bottom and sides of the mortar completely with the foil, preventing sample loss. Create a lip in one side the foil for later pouring of tissue into a 1.5 mL tube. Pour a small amount of liquid nitrogen from a small tabletop dewar into the mortar to cool it. Place the pestle inside the mortar and into the remaining liquid nitrogen to cool. Before the liquid nitrogen evaporates, place 10–20 mg of the frozen sample (this is specific for skeletal muscle tissue) into the mortar and grind the tissue under liquid nitrogen with the motor and pestle in order to create a homogenous sample. Creating a homogenous sample for DNA isolation is critical, especially with tissue samples such as skeletal muscle, as tissues, including different tissue regions, will contain different cellular types as well as cells within different growth phases. However, it should be noted that in vitro samples similarly contain cells in various growth phases unless treated appropriately beforehand. Nucleosome mapping has been accomplished in both in vitro and in vivo samples using similar methods such as outlined here [29, 30, 33, 34] and Fig. 1. Once the tissue sample is crushed into small pieces, remove the foil square containing the sample and liquid nitrogen from the mortar and pour the remaining liquid nitrogen and ground tissue sample into a 1.5 mL tube. If the liquid nitrogen evaporates before completion of this step, pour more liquid nitrogen into the mortar from a small tabletop dewar being careful not to create too much pressure from the pouring to prevent sample loss. You may also scrape any remaining ground sample from the foil with a spatula into the 1.5 mL tube if necessary. Allow any excess liquid nitrogen to evaporate from the 1.5 mL tube and add 0.5 mL of 0.25 M sucrose buffer into the 1.5 mL tube. Place the tube on ice. Remove the foil from the mortar and discard. Repeat for all samples.

3.4.2 Nuclear and Chromatin Isolation

To isolate nuclei from the sample, homogenize the ground tissue with 0.25 M sucrose buffer in a 1 mL Dounce homogenizer on ice. Take 1.5 mL tube containing the ground sample plus sucrose buffer

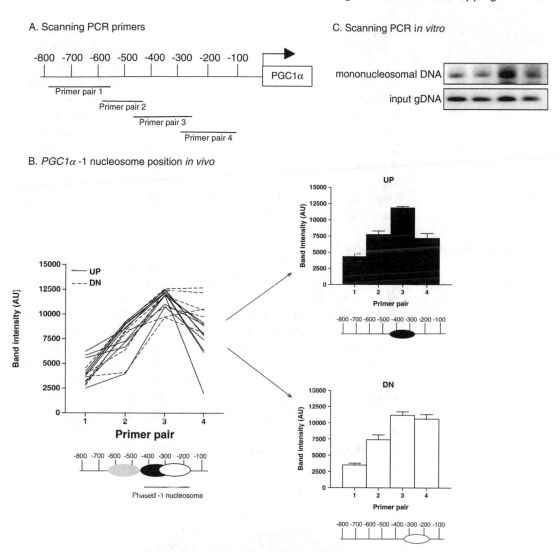

Fig. 1 Scanning PCR in vivo and in vitro. (**a**) qPCR primers are designed to target a specific genomic locus, here the promoter region directly upstream of the transcriptional start site in the gene *PGC1α*. Primer pairs typically targeting the -1 nucleosome position, as seen here, span a region of the gene. In our studies, the forward primer of one pair is the reverse primer (in the reverse complement) in the adjacent pair, creating the overlap to determine nucleosome position. (**b**) In our recent study, overlapping primer pairs in A were used to map the -1 nucleosome in *PGC1α* in in vivo skeletal muscle samples [29]. Resulting qPCR amplicons were run on a 1.5% agarose gel and band intensities were measured via densitometry using ImageJ sofware. Results are shown for each individual sample in the line graph as arbitary units (AU). Based on the band intensity, nucleosome position was inferred for samples and depicted under the line graph. Two populations of samples were seen in our data, resulting in separation of samples into two treatment groups, one having the -1 nucleosome further upstream (UP) from the transcriptional start site and one group exhibiting the -1 nucleosome farther downstream (DN). (**c**) -1 nucleosome mapping was performed similarly in vitro, using primary myocyte samples extracted from muscle of lean and obese individuals and cultured. Cells were treated with a PFI (pioglitazone, forskolin, and inositol) cocktail to mimic exercise training in vitro. qPCR results were run on a 1.5% agarose gel and are shown only for the primer pair exhibiting differential nucleosome occupancy in the samples

and mix by flicking or inverting to resuspend the tissue into solution. Pour the buffer and tissue into a cold 1 mL Dounce homogenizer on ice. Place the empty 1.5 mL tube on ice. Homogenize the tissue sample 5–6× while on ice or until no pieces of tissue are visible. Quickly pour the homogenized sample back into the cold 1.5 mL tube. Add an additional 0.5 mL of 0.25 M sucrose buffer into the 1.5 mL tube, giving a final volume close to 1 mL. Centrifuge the homogenate at 4 °C, 10 min, 6000×g. Remove and discard the supernatant by pipetting it off. Wash the pellet with 1 mL sucrose buffer. Centrifuge at 4 °C, 20 min, 14,000×g. Discard the supernatant and resuspend the pellet in 1 mL digestion buffer to release the native chromatin from the nuclei (see Sect. 4).

3.4.3 Mononucleosomal DNA Fragmentation and Purification

Aliquot 0.5 mL of each sample into 1.5 mL tubes. Into tube 1, add 0.67 μL of MNase (20 U MNase). Do nothing to tube 2 (see Sect.4). Of note, tube 1 will now contain MNase-digested mononucleosomal DNA and tube 2 will contain undigested, genomic DNA (gDNA) to be used as an input control in the scanning PCR. Incubate samples for 15 min at 37 °C (for digestion into mononucleosomal fragments in tube 1). Incubation times and amounts of MNase will vary based on the amount and type of sample used (see Sect. 4; Fig. 2). Stop the MNase digestion by adding 12.5 μL of 0.2 M EDTA (5 mM final concentration) to each 500 μL sample and mixing by flicking. Promptly place samples on ice, and incubate on ice for 5 min. Centrifuge samples for 5 min at 8000×g. Discard the supernatant and resuspend the pel-

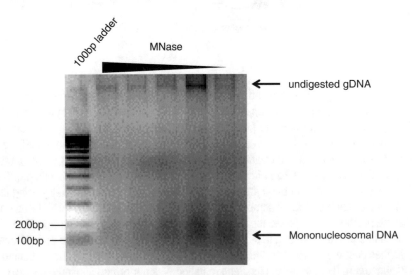

Fig. 2 MNase titration with 10 mg of skeletal muscle. Mononucleosomal DNA was extracted from 10 mg of skeletal muscle following the protocol outlined in the chapter. Each 10 mg sample was treated with a varying concentration of MNase during the digestion step to determine the optimal dose used to generate at least 95 % digestion of gDNA into mononucleosomal DNA fragments

let in 200 μL of lysis buffer. Pipette up and down to mix and vortex to lyse. Add 20 μL of 1 mg/mL proteinase K to each tube and incubate overnight in a heat block set at 37 °C to digest histone proteins from the mononucleosomal DNA. Samples may be used immediately or may be stored at −20 °C short term or −80 °C long term for later analyses. Purify the mononucleosomal DNA and gDNA by ethanol precipitation.

3.5 Scanning qPCR

Overlapping primer pairs (see Fig. 1a) should be designed to cover the genomic locus of interest, such as the promoter region containing the -1 nucleosome, which typically spans from the -800 nucleotide to the +200 nucleotide and encompasses the transcriptional start site. Primer pairs should be designed following guidelines for any general PCR reaction, and targeting amplification of a 150–200 bp region. For each primer pair, mononucleosomal and gDNA samples should be run in at least duplicate and preferably in triplicate using general PCR settings according to your PCR master mix and primer pair melting temperatures. The amount of template DNA may vary depending on your PCR platform. Generally, 15 ng of mononucleosomal DNA and 3 ng of gDNA is adequate for scanning qPCR. Run PCR products for both mononucleosomal and gDNA samples on a 1.5% agarose gel and visualize using a gel imager or UV lamp. Measure band densities using a software program, such as MacBiophotonics ImageJ (Bethesda, MD). Divide mononucleosomal band intensity by the intensity of the corresponding input gDNA. Graph results and run appropriate statistics to determine differential positioning or occupancy for each primer pair/genomic locus. For example, amplification in sample 1 with primer pair 2 but not primer pair 3, coupled with absence of amplification in sample 2 with primer pair 2 but amplification with primer pair 3 may indicate nucleosome repositioning in sample 2 compared to sample 1. Amplification in samples 1 and 2 with primer pair 4, but with higher band intensity in sample 2 compared to 1 would indicate differences in nucleosome occupancy at this locus.

4 Notes

The method outlined here for scanning PCR, using mononucleosomal DNA and qPCR, has worked successfully and reproducibly in both skeletal muscle tissue samples and myocyte (primary and immortalized) cell samples within our laboratory. Additionally, this method has been employed by others for nucleosome mapping of specific genomic loci [35]. It should be noted that all nucleosome mapping results, whether via scanning PCR, MNase-seq, primer extension, etc. should be validated by measuring corresponding gene expression of the gene of interest via qRT-PCR. Although some investigators choose to fix tissues and cells prior to mononucleosomal DNA isolation in an effort to prevent spurious results due to the DNA isolation [35, 36], others have found that fixing tissue and cells prior to mononucleosomal DNA isolation may lead to misidentification of nucleosome-bound regions, as fixation results in binding of histone, as well as other, proteins to the gDNA [37, 38]. In the latter case, subsequent digestion by MNase may lead to identification not only of nucleosomal regions but also of regions where transcription factors and other regulatory proteins may have been bound [39]. Here, we prefer the former method devoid of fixation, favoring native DNA for nucleosome mapping, as we assume that with all samples being treated equally during extraction, any differential results found in nucleosome positioning and occupancy are most likely due to our treatment effect.

As mentioned previously, this method can be modified for use in cells. This modification calls for omission of **steps 3–9**, with cells being processed directly after collecting, pelleting and removing medium. Within the literature [34, 35, 40] and in our efforts, one may find that different sample types, here tissues vs. cells, may require alteration of either the dose of MNase or the time of MNase digestion to prevent under- or overdigestion of the gDNA into mononucleosomal fragments. Thus, we recommend when performing these methods on a new sample type, to do a dose– or time–response using at least three concentrations of MNase or three MNase digestion times during the MNase digestion step (**step 16**) and running all products on an agarose. 95 % digestion of the gDNA into a fragment of approximately 175 bp is adequate digestion for qPCR and nucleosome mapping (Fig. 2). We have also observed that in performing our triplicate replication of samples during the qPCR, if varying results in band intensities are observed for the same sample, the final product from the mononucleosomal DNA digestion may not be completely free of salts or detergents which may interfere with PCR amplification. If this occurs, ethanol precipitation is recommended for the sample. Column and gel purification of samples generally results in too much sample loss. Alternatively, a more robust DNA polymerase may be required for your scanning qPCR reaction. Mononucleosomal and genomic DNA from this isolation procedure can be used in downstream qRT-PCR in lieu of qPCR as an alternative approach to nucleosome mapping of targeted genomic loci if preferred by the researcher [41].

Using either qPCR or qRT-PCR of mononucleosomal and genomic DNA samples with overlapping primers pairs, as outlined here, is sufficient to determine nucleosome positioning and occupancy at target genomic loci and may help us determine those loci that are epigenetically regulated at the onset and during the progression of disease.

References

1. Suzuki MM, Bird A (2008) DNA methylation landscapes: provocative insights from epigenomics. Nat Rev Genet 9(6):465–476. doi:10.1038/nrg2341

2. Ropero S, Esteller M (2007) The role of histone deacetylases (HDACs) in human cancer. Mol Oncol 1:19–25. doi:10.1016/j.molonc.2007.01.001

3. Chuang JC, Jones PA (2007) Epigenetics and MicroRNAs. Pediatr Res 61:24R–29R. doi:10.1203/pdr.0b013e3180457684

4. Margueron R, Reinberg D (2010) Chromatin structure and the inheritance of epigenetic information. Nat Rev Genet 11:285–296. doi:10.1038/nrg2752

5. Schones DE, Cui K, Cuddapah S, Roh TY, Barski A, Wang Z, Wei G, Zhao K (2008) Dynamic regulation of nucleosome positioning in the human genome. Cell 132(5):887–898. doi:10.1016/j.cell.2008.02.022

6. Segal E, Widom J (2009) What controls nucleosome positions? Trends Genet 25(8):335–343. doi:10.1016/j.tig.2009.06.002

7. Zentner GE, Henikoff S (2013) Regulation of nucleosome dynamics by histone modifications. Nat Struct Mol Biol 20(3):259–266. doi:10.1038/nsmb.2470

8. Chandrasekharan MB, Huang F, Sun ZW (2009) Ubiquitination of histone H2B regulates chromatin dynamics by enhancing nucleosome stability. Proc Natl Acad Sci U S A 106:16686–16691. doi:10.1073/pnas.0907862106, Epub 2009 Sep 10

9. Nowak SJ, Corces VG (2004) Phosphorylation of histone H3: a balancing act between chromosome condensation and transcriptional activation. Trends Genet 20(4):214–220. doi:10.1016/j.tig.2004.02.007, http://dx.doi.org/

10. Radman-Livaja M, Rando OJ (2010) Nucleosome positioning: how is it established, and why does it matter? Dev Biol 339(2):258–266. doi:10.1016/j.ydbio.2009.06.012

11. Workman JL, Kingston RE (1998) Alteration of nucleosome structure as a mechanism of transcriptional regulation. Annu Rev Biochem 67:545–579. doi:10.1146/annurev.biochem.67.1.545

12. Whitehouse I, Rando OJ, Delrow J, Tsukiyama T (2007) Chromatin remodelling at promoters suppresses antisense transcription. Nature 450(7172):1031–1035. doi:10.1038/nature06391

13. Henikoff S (2008) Nucleosome destabilization in the epigenetic regulation of gene expression. Nat Rev Genet 9(1):15–26. doi:10.1038/nrg2206

14. Hogan GJ, Lee CK, Lieb JD (2006) Cell cycle-specified fluctuation of nucleosome occupancy at gene promoters. PLoS Genet 2(9):e158. doi:10.1371/journal.pgen.0020158

15. Shivaswamy S, Bhinge A, Zhao Y, Jones S, Hirst M, Iyer VR (2008) Dynamic remodeling of individual nucleosomes across a eukaryotic genome in response to transcriptional perturbation. PLoS Biol 6(3):e65. doi:10.1371/journal.pbio.0060065

16. Jiang C, Pugh BF (2009) A compiled and systematic reference map of nucleosome positions across the Saccharomyces cerevisiae genome. Genome Biol 10(10):R109. doi:10.1186/gb-2009-10-10-r109

17. Zhao X, Pendergrast PS, Hernandez N (2001) A positioned nucleosome on the human U6 promoter allows recruitment of SNAPc by the Oct-1 POU domain. Mol Cell 7(3):539–549

18. Khorasanizadeh S (2004) The nucleosome: from genomic organization to genomic regulation. Cell 116:259–272

19. Peckham HE, Thurman RE, Fu Y, Stamatoyannopoulos JA, Noble WS, Struhl K, Weng Z (2007) Nucleosome positioning signals in genomic DNA. Genome Res 17(8):1170–1177. doi:10.1101/gr.6101007

20. Hartley PD, Madhani HD (2009) Mechanisms that specify promoter nucleosome location and identity. Cell 137(3):445–458. doi:10.1016/j.cell.2009.02.043

21. Workman JL, Kingston RE (1992) Nucleosome core displacement in vitro via a metastable transcription factor-nucleosome complex. Science 258(5089):1780–1784

22. Mollazadeh-Beidokhti L, Deseigne J, Lacoste D, Mohammad-Rafiee F, Schiessel H (2009) Stochastic model for nucleosome sliding under an external force. Phys Rev E Stat Nonlin Soft Matter Phys 79(3 Pt 1):031922

23. Lin JC, Jeong S, Liang G, Takai D, Fatemi M, Tsai YC, Egger G, Gal-Yam EN, Jones PA (2007) Role of nucleosomal occupancy in the epigenetic silencing of the MLH1 CpG island. Cancer Cell 12(5):432–444. doi:10.1016/j.ccr.2007.10.014

24. Morey L, Brenner C, Fazi F, Villa R, Gutierrez A, Buschbeck M, Nervi C, Minucci S, Fuks F, Croce LD (2008) MBD3, a component of the

NuRD complex facilitates chromatin alteration and deposition of epigenetic marks. Mol Cell Biol 28(19):5912–5923. doi:10.1128/MCB.00467-08

25. Jones S, Wang TL, Shih Ie M, Mao TL, Nakayama K, Roden R, Glas R, Slamon D, Diaz LA, Vogelstein B, Kinzler KW, Velculescu VE, Papadopoulos N (2010) Frequent mutations of chromatin remodeling gene ARID1A in ovarian clear cell carcinoma. Science 330(6001):228–231. doi:10.1126/science.1196333

26. Pinney SE, Simmons RA (2010) Epigenetic mechanisms in the development of type 2 diabetes. Trends Endocrinol Metab 21:223–229. doi:10.1016/j.tem.2009.10.002, Epub 2009 Oct 26

27. Campion J, Milagro FI, Martinez JA (2009) Individuality and epigenetics in obesity. Obes Rev 10:383–392. doi:10.1111/j.1467-789X.2009.00595.x, Epub 2009 Apr 21

28. de Mello VD, Pulkkinen L, Lalli M, Kolehmainen M, Pihlajamaki J, Uusitupa M (2014) DNA methylation in obesity and type 2 diabetes. Ann Med 46:103–113. doi:10.3109/07853890.2013.857259, Epub 2014 Apr 30

29. Henagan TM, Stewart LK, Forney LA, Sparks LM, Johannsen N, Church TS (2014) PGC1α -1 nucleosome position and splice variant expression and cardiovascular disease risk in overweight and obese individuals. PPAR Res 2014:895734. doi:10.1155/2014/895734

30. Henagan TM, Stefanska B, Fang Z, Navard AM, Ye J, Lenard NR, Devarshi PP (2015) Sodium butyrate epigenetically modulates high-fat diet-induced skeletal muscle mitochondrial adaptation, obesity and insulin resistance through nucleosome positioning. Br J Pharmacol 172(11):2782–2798. doi:10.1111/bph.13058

31. Drake AJ, McPherson RC, Godfrey KM, Cooper C, Lillycrop KA, Hanson MA, Meehan RR, Seckl JR, Reynolds RM (2012) An unbalanced maternal diet in pregnancy associates with offspring epigenetic changes in genes controlling glucocorticoid action and foetal growth. Clin Endocrinol (Oxf) 77(6):808–815.doi:10.1111/j.1365-2265.2012.04453.x

32. Aagaard-Tillery KM, Grove K, Bishop J, Ke X, Fu Q, McKnight R, Lane RH (2008) Developmental origins of disease and determi-nants of chromatin structure: maternal diet modifies the primate fetal epigenome. J Mol Endocrinol 41(2):91–102. doi:10.1677/jme-08-0025

33. Infante J, Law GL, Young E (2012) Analysis of nucleosome positioning using a nucleosome-scanning assay. In: Morse RH (ed) Chromatin remodeling, vol 833, Methods Mol Biol. Humana, New York, pp 63–87. doi:10.1007/978-1-61779-477-3_5

34. Sekinger EA, Moqtaderi Z, Struhl K (2005) Intrinsic histone-DNA interactions and low nucleosome density are important for preferential accessibility of promoter regions in yeast. Mol Cell 18(6):735–748. doi:10.1016/j.molcel.2005.05.003, http://dx.doi.org/

35. Creamer KM, Job G, Shanker S, Neale GA, Lin Y, Bartholomew B, Partridge JF (2014) The Mi-2 homolog Mit1 actively positions nucleosomes within heterochromatin to suppress transcription. Mol Cell Biol 34:2046–2061. doi:10.1128/mcb.01609-13

36. Mavrich TN, Ioshikhes IP, Venters BJ, Jiang C, Tomsho LP, Qi J, Schuster SC, Albert I, Pugh BF (2008) A barrier nucleosome model for statistical positioning of nucleosomes throughout the yeast genome. Genome Res 18:1073–1083. doi:10.1101/gr.078261.108, Epub 2008 Jun 12

37. Clark DJ (2010) Nucleosome positioning, nucleosome spacing and the nucleosome code. J Biomol Struct Dyn 27:781–793. doi:10.1080/073911010010524945

38. Fragoso G, John S, Roberts MS, Hager GL (1995) Nucleosome positioning on the MMTV LTR results from the frequency-biased occupancy of multiple frames. Genes Dev 9:1933–1947

39. Boeger H, Griesenbeck J, Strattan JS, Kornberg RD (2003) Nucleosomes unfold completely at a transcriptionally active promoter. Mol Cell 11:1587–1598

40. Sebeson A, Xi L, Zhang Q, Sigmund A, Wang JP, Widom J, Wang X (2015) Differential nucleosome occupancies across Oct4-Sox2 binding sites in murine embryonic stem cells. PLoS One 10:e0127214. doi:10.1371/journal.pone.0127214, eCollection 2015

41. Infante JJ, Law GL, Young ET (2012) Analysis of nucleosome positioning using a nucleosome-scanning assay. Methods Mol Biol 833:63–87. doi:10.1007/978-1-61779-477-3_5

Chapter 5

Synthesis and Application of Cell-Permeable Metabolites for Modulating Chromatin Modifications Regulated by α-Ketoglutarate-Dependent Enzymes

Hunter T. Balduf, Antonella Pepe, and Ann L. Kirchmaier

Abstract

Direct links between altered metabolism, dysregulation of epigenetic processes, and cancer have been established via investigation of cancer- and syndrome-associated mutations in genes encoding key enzymes of intermediary metabolism. Here, we provide an outline for the synthesis of cell-permeable forms of the cellular metabolites (R)-2-hydroxyglutarate and (L)-2-hydroxyglutarate, and their application for the inhibition of α-ketoglutarate-dependent Jumonji histone demethylases.

Key words α-ketoglutarate, (R)-2-hydroxyglutarate, (L)-2-hydroxyglutarate, Cancer, Leukemia, Glioma, Epigenetics, Histone methylation

1 Introduction

Genome-wide alterations in histone methylation and DNA modification patterns are commonly associated with changes to chromatin structure and composition at genes or their regulatory regions, as well as alterations in gene expression. In cancers of the hematopoietic, glial and other cell lineages, such changes to the epigenome are often linked to mutations in genes encoding enzymes involved in regulating histone or DNA methylation ([1–4], and references within). Cancers derived from these cell lineages are often alternatively associated with mutations in several metabolic enzymes, leading to perturbations in cellular metabolism and the accumulation of "oncometabolites." Accumulation of two such metabolites, (R)-2-hydroxyglutarate (R2HG) and (L)-2-hydroxyglutarate (L2HG), results in the inhibition of several members of Jumonji family of histone demethylases as well as the Tet family of oxygenases, and are predicted to perturb epigenetic processes in a manner that partly phenocopies that of mutations in the chromatin modifying

Barbara Stefanska and David J. MacEwan (eds.), *Epigenetics and Gene Expression in Cancer, Inflammatory and Immune Diseases*, Methods in Pharmacology and Toxicology, DOI 10.1007/978-1-4939-6743-8_5, © Springer Science+Business Media LLC 2017

enzymes themselves [5–8]. This metabolite-mediated inhibition leads to increased cellular histone methylation levels via preventing histone demethylation. Metabolite-mediated inhibition also leads to reduced 5-hydroxymethylcytosine (5hmC) levels in DNA via blocking Tet-dependent conversion of 5-methylcytosine (5mC) to 5hmC [5–8].

The *de novo* establishment of DNA methylation patterns may also be adversely influenced by oncometabolite-dependent changes to histone methylation. DNA methyltransferase DNMT3A activity is regulated via histone methylation-status dependent interactions with the N-terminal tail of histone H3 [9–11]. In addition, both passive loss and active removal of DNA methylation is likely affected in cells with elevated levels of R2HG or L2HG through the inactivation of Tet oxygenases. DNA binding of the maintenance methyltransferase complex UHRF1/DNMT1 is inhibited by 5hmC [12, 13]. During active removal of DNA methylation, Tet oxygenase-dependent conversion of 5mC to 5hmC, then to 5-formylcytosine (5fC), and next to 5-carboxylcytosine (5caC) enables the subsequent replacement of 5fC and 5caC with C by DNA glycosylase during base excision repair [14–17]. Alternatively, 5hmC may be converted to 5-hydroxymethyluridine (5-hmU) by AID/APOBEC enzymes, and then removed during base excision repair [18]. Currently, much work remains to identify key chromosomal locations where perturbations to chromatin in the presence of oncometabolites are directly contributing to oncogenesis.

Below, we briefly outline current understanding of cellular pathways associated with the metabolism of R2HG and L2HG, and highlight several links between R2HG or L2HG and epigenetic processes.

(R)-2-Hydroxyglutarate (R2HG): During normal metabolism, vR2HG is generated during degradation of hydroxylysine [19] or 5-aminolevulinate, and additional routes [20]. In a process sometimes referred to as "metabolic repair," R2HG can be converted to α-ketoglutarate (α-KG) by D-2-hydroxyglutarate dehydrogenase (DHGDH; D-lactate dehydrogenase) [21–23]. Although normal physiological role(s) of R2HG remain poorly understood, mutations that disrupt the activity of the metabolic repair enzyme DHGDH or that confer novel activities to cytoplasmic/mitochondrial isocitrate dehydrogenases (IDH1 and IDH2) lead to the accumulation of high levels of R2HG in cells, result in metabolic disorders, and alter epigenetic processes. Although wild-type IDH1 and IDH2 normally convert isocitrate to α-KG during the Krebs (TCA) cycle (Fig. 1), neomorphic IDH mutants instead convert α-KG to R2HG [24], resulting in elevated cellular levels of R2HG [24–27] (Fig. 1). Such neomorphic mutants are commonly found in neoplasms ranging from gliomas, T cell lymphomas and cholangiocarcinomas to acute myeloid leukemia [24, 26–32].

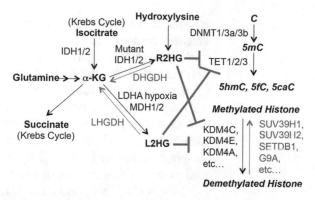

Fig. 1 R2HG ((R)-2-hydroxyglutarate) and L2HG ((L)-2-hydroxyglutarate) in Metabolism. Metabolites (*bold*); modification states (*bold + italics*). *IDH1/2* Isocitrate dehydrogenases, *LHGDH* L-2-Hydroxyglutarate dehydrogenase, *DHGDH* D-2-Hydroxyglutarate dehydrogenase, *LDHA* Lactate dehydrogenase, *MDH1/2* Malate dehydrogenases, *DNMT1/3a/3b* DNA methyltransferases, *TET1/2/3* Tet oxygenases, *KDM4C/E/A* etc. Jumonji domain-containing histone demethylases, *SUV39H1/H2, SETDB1, G9A* histone methyltransferases, *C* unmethylated DNA, *5mC* methylated DNA, *5hmC* hydroxymethylated DNA, *5fC* 5-formylcytosine in DNA, *5caC* 5-carboxylcytosine in DNA

These mutations alter the substrate-binding pocket of IDH1/2, and IDH1 requires the presence of wild-type IDH to synthesize the oncometabolite, whereas IDH2 does not [33–35].

R2HG itself binds within the catalytic site of several α-KG-dependent enzymes involved in epigenetic processes. R2HG can inhibit the activity of histone demethylases to varying degrees, including KDM4E [5], KDM4C, and KDM4A [6]. R2HG also inhibits α-KG-dependent Tet oxygenases [7, 8], and, thus, can alter 5mC and 5hmC levels in chromosomal DNA (Fig. 1). Physiological levels of R2HG can modulate chromatin modifications, and gliomas with IDH1/IDH2 mutations have lower levels of 5hmC than their normal counterparts [8]. Also, consistent with a direct association between elevated R2HG levels and oncogenesis, exposure to a cell permeable form of R2HG promotes leukemic transformation *in vitro* [36].

(L)-2-Hydroxyglutarate (L2HG): Like R2HG, the metabolite L2HG also inhibits Jumonji histone demethylases as well as Tet oxygenases [5–8] (Fig. 1), and accumulation of L2HG in cells correlates with a decrease in 5hmC and an increase in histone methylation [37]. Under certain environmental conditions, L2HG is thought to play a role in helping to maintain cellular homeostasis and regulate energy metabolism through inhibition of glycolysis and oxygen consumption. In metabolism, Malate dehydrogenases (MDH1 and MDH2) and Lactate dehydrogenase (LDHA) produce L2HG directly from α-KG [38–41]. Although all three

enzymes contribute to the synthesis of L2HG, LDHA is the major enzyme responsible for the accumulation of L2HG specifically during hypoxia [41], and this accumulated L2HG acts as an antagonist of the α-KG-dependent prolylhydroxylase EglN, a regulator of the hypoxia-inducible transcription factor HIF1 [36, 42]. Through metabolic repair, L2HG can be converted to α-KG by L-2-Hydroxyglutarate dehydrogenase (LHGDH) [41] (Fig. 1). Mutations in LHGDH lead to accumulation of L2HG and metabolic disorder (e.g., L-2-hydroxyglutaric aciduria [21, 43]) as well as reduced 5hmC levels [37].

Like R2HG, accumulation of L2HG has been observed in cancer; L2HG is commonly elevated in renal cancer, in part, through the loss of LHGDH [37, 44]. However, despite typically being a more potent inhibitor of chromatin modifying enzymes than R2HG [6, 8, 42], thus far L2HG has been less frequently linked to cancer than R2HG [36]. This difference has been proposed to be related to the role of L2HG as an antagonist to EglN. In contrast, R2HG serves as an agonist of EglN [36, 42].

Here, we provide strategies for the syntheses of cell-permeable forms of R2HG and L2HG, octyl-R-2-hydroxyglutarate (octyl-R2HG) and octyl-L-2-hydroxyglutarate (octyl-L2HG), their application for modulating histone methylation in cell culture and subsequent analysis of histone methylation levels by immunoblotting. For additional information on the synthesis and application of octyl-R2HG or octyl-L2HG to modulate histone methylation or DNA hydroxymethylation levels, or for the analyses of hypoxia/normoxia, please also *see*, e.g., [6, 37, 45–48].

2   Materials

2.1   Synthesis of Octyl-R-2-hydroxyglutarate or Octyl-L-2-hydroxyglutarate

Anhydrous sodium sulfate (Aldrich #SX0760), D-glutamic acid (Aldrich #G1001), L-glutamic acid (Aldrich #G1251), benzyl alcohol (Aldrich #24122), tetrafluoroboric acid diethyl ether complex (Aldrich #400068), activated charcoal (Aldrich #242276), ethyl acetate (Macron, ACS grade, #4992), sodium nitrite (Aldrich #237213), acetic acid (Macron #V193-45), double distilled water, dimethylformamide (Aldrich #227056), potassium bicarbonate (Amresco #0889), 1-iodooctane (Aldrich #238295), hexanes (Fisher #H292-20), methanol (Fisher #A452-4), hydrogen, palladium on carbon (Aldrich #205699), celite (Alfa Aesar #B22658), dichloromethane (Macron #4879-10).

Silica gel columns (Yamazen Corporation, silica gel 30 μm, 60 Å, dimensions of 40 g columns 2.6 ID×12.4 cm packed length; 16 g columns 2.0 ID×8.4 cm packed length, 7 g columns 1.6 ID×7.0 cm packed length).

Büchi Rotavapor Model R-215 or equivalent rotary evaporator.

Separatory funnel.

TLC plates: silica gel 60 F254 on aluminum support (Merck).

Buchner-type filtration funnel with sintered disc, and connection for vacuum.

Automated purification system: Yamazen Smart Flash EPCLC W-Prep 2XY with UV detector and fraction collector, or equivalent.

NMR spectrometer: Bruker AV500HD (500 MHz) NMR spectrometer equipped with a 5 mm BBFO Z-gradient cryoprobe Prodigy, or equivalent. Proton chemical shifts are reported in ppm (δ) relative to the solvent reference relative to tetramethylsilane (TMS) (CDCl3, δ 7.26). Data are reported as follows: chemical shift (multiplicity [singlet (s), doublet (d), triplet (t), quartet (q) and multiplet (m)], coupling constants [Hz], integration). Carbon NMR spectra were recorded with complete proton decoupling. Carbon chemical shifts were reported in ppm (δ) relative to TMS, with the respective solvent resonance as the internal standard (CDCl$_3$, δ 77.0).

Reverse phase HPLC: Agilent 1200 HPLC, equipped with diode array detector and Chiralpack IC 3 column (3 µm, 46 mm, 100 mm) or equivalent. The conditions used are as follows: flow rate = 0.8 ml/min; Solvent A = water + 0.01 % TFA; Solvent B = acetonitrile. At 0 min 60 % B, at 10 min 65 % B, at 15 min 60 % B.

Mass spectrometry: Agilent MSD/TOF, coupled with an Agilent 1100HPLC system, with autosampler and photodiode array (PDA) detector or equivalent.

2.2 Cell Culture and Treatment with Octyl-R-2-hydroxyglutarate or Octyl-L-2-hydroxyglutarate

Appropriate cell line and tissue culture medium: Chronic Myelogenous Leukemia cell line K-562 (ATCC #CCL-243), Iscove's Modified Dulbecco's Medium, IMDM, with L-glutamine and 25 mM HEPES (Gibco #12200-036) containing 100 U/ml penicillin, 100 mg/ml streptomycin (Gibco #15140-122 or equivalent) and 10 % fetal bovine serum (FBS).

1× phosphate buffered saline (PBS): 137 mM NaCl, 2.7 mM KCl, 10 mM Na$_2$HPO$_4$, 1.8 mM KH$_2$PO$_4$. Adjust to pH 7.4 and filter through a 0.2 µm filter.

0.25 % trypsin–EDTA (Gibco BRL #25200-056 or equivalent).

0.4 % (w/v) Trypan Blue.

60 mm tissue culture dishes.

15 ml conical tubes, 1.5 ml microfuge tubes.

Hemocytometer.

Centrifuge.

37 °C CO_2 humidified incubator.

Biosafety cabinet.

2.3 Mammalian Whole Cell Extracts

0.2 M phenylmethanesulfonyl fluoride (PMSF) in 100 % ethanol, store at −80 °C.

Extraction Buffer: 50 mM Tris–HCl pH 7.4, 150 mM NaCl, 1 % NP-40 (v/v), 0.25 % Na-deoxycholate. Store at 4 °C.

15 ml conical tubes, 1.5 ml microfuge tubes.

Centrifuge.

Microcentrifuge.

Branson Sonifier 450 sonicator or equivalent.

2.4 Protein Blotting

1× PBS, distilled H_2O, methanol.

Gel electrophoresis: Stock solutions of 30 % acrylamide–bis 29:1, 1 M Tris–HCl, pH 8.8, 1 M Tris–HCl, pH 6.8, 20 % (w/v) sodium dodecyl sulfate (SDS), 10 % (w/v) ammonium persulfate (APS), tetramethylethylenediamine (TEMED), butanol.

SDS-PAGE Running Buffer: 25 mM Tris base pH 8.8, 190 mM glycine, 0.1 % SDS. Adjust to pH 8.3.

4× Loading Buffer: 0.25 M Tris–HCl, pH 6.8, 8 % SDS, 30 % glycerol, 0.1 % (w/v) bromophenol blue. Store at 4 °C. Add β-mercaptoethanol to 10 % final concentration in 4× Loading buffer immediately prior to use.

Protein Molecular Weight Ladder (PAGE Ruler, Thermo Fisher, #26616 or equivalent).

Transfer Buffer: 25 mM Tris Base pH 8.8, 190 mM glycine, 20 % methanol. Adjust to pH 8.3. Chill to 4 °C prior to use.

Protein Blots: PVDF Membrane (Bio-Rad #162-0177 or equivalent), Whatman paper (GE Health Sciences #GB003 or equivalent), rabbit polyclonal anti-histone H3K79me2 antibodies (Upstate #07-366), rabbit polyclonal anti-histone H3 antibodies (Abcam # ab1791), donkey polyclonal anti-rabbit IgG-HRP antibodies (GE Healthcare, #NA934), Luminata Crescendo Western HRP Substrate (EMD Millipore, #WBLUR0500), or equivalent.

PBST: 1× PBS, 0.1 % Tween 20. Store at 4 °C.

Blocking Buffer: 4 % (w/v) Powdered Milk (Meijer instant nonfat powdered milk or equivalent) in PBST. Store at 4 °C.

0.2 M NaOH.

15 ml conical tubes, 1.5 ml microfuge tubes.

Bio-Rad Mini-Protean Electrophoresis Tetra Cell System or equivalent.

Bio-Rad ChemiDoc XRS+ or equivalent.

3   Methods

3.1 Synthesis of Octyl-R-2-hydroxyglutarate

(For the synthesis of octyl-L-2-hydroxyglutarate, follow the protocol for octyl-R-2-hydroxyglutarate outlined below in Sects. 3.1.1–3.1.3, except use L-glutamic acid in **step 2** of Sect. 3.1.1; *see* Fig. 2 and **Note 1**).

3.1.1 Synthesis of (R)-2-amino-5-(benzyloxy)-5-oxopentanoic Acid

Schema for synthesis of (R)-2-amino-5-(benzyloxy)-5-oxopentanoic acid from benzyl alcohol and D-glutamic acid is shown in Fig. 2, top panel.

1. Add 2.00 g anhydrous sodium sulfate (14.1 mmol) to a two-necked flame dried round-bottom flask equipped with a magnetic stirring bar, a nitrogen inlet adapter connected to a nitrogen/vacuum manifold and a rubber septum.

2. Add 2.00 g D-glutamic acid (13.6 mmol) to the flask evacuate and back-fill the flask with nitrogen three times and add 25.0 ml benzyl alcohol.

3. Add 3.70 ml tetrafluoroboric acid diethyl ether complex dropwise (27.2 mmol) and stir at room temperature for 15 h, then add 75.0 ml of anhydrous THF to the milky white suspension.

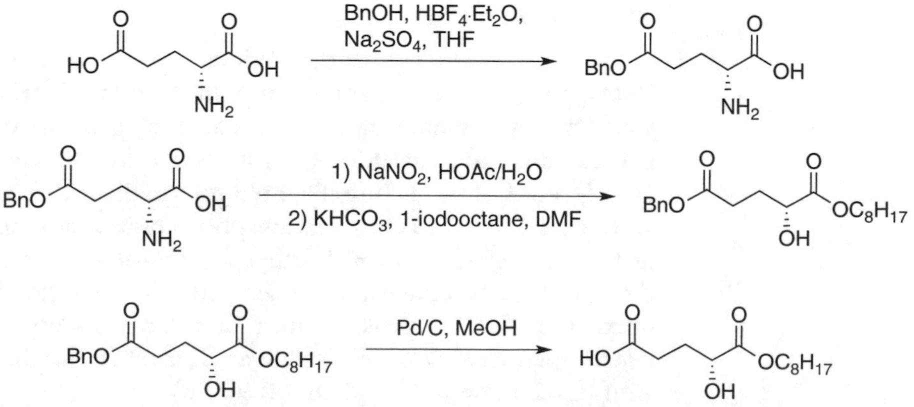

Fig. 2 Synthesis of octyl-R-2-hydroxyglutarate, octyl-R2HG. Schema for synthesis of (R)-2-amino-5-(benzyloxy)-5-oxopentanoic acid from benzyl alcohol and D-glutamic acid (*top panel*; Sect. 3.1.1); synthesis of 5-benzyl 1-octyl (R)-2-hydroxypentanedioate from (R)-2-amino-5-(benzyloxy)-5-oxopentanoic acid (*middle panel*; Sect. 3.1.2); synthesis of (R)-4-hydroxy-5-(octyloxy)-5-oxopentanoic acid from 5-benzyl 1-octyl (R)-2-hydroxypentanedioate (*bottom panel*; Sect. 3.1.3). Schema for synthesis of the L enantiomer, octyl-L2HG, is analogous, except L-glutamic acid is used instead of D-glutamic acid (*see* Sect. 3.1 and **Note1**).

4. Pour a pad of activated charcoal (as a slurry in anhydrous THF) to a glass Buchner-type filtration funnel with sintered disc, and connection for vacuum. Filter the reaction mixture through this pad of charcoal, then add 4.10 ml triethyl amine to the clear filtrate.

5. Triturate the resulting white slurry with ethyl acetate (100.0 ml) and filter the mixture on a glass Buchner-type filtration funnel with sintered disc, and connection for vacuum to isolate the title compound as granular colorless solid (~78% yield, ~2.50 g).

3.1.2 Synthesis of 5-benzyl 1-octyl (R)-2-hydroxy-pentanedioate

Schema for synthesis of 5-benzyl 1-octyl (R)-2-hydroxypentanedioate from (R)-2-amino-5-(benzyloxy)-5-oxopentanoic acid is shown in Fig. 2, middle panel.

1. Resuspend 1.48 g (R)-2-amino-5-(benzyloxy)-5-oxopentanoic acid (6.24 mmol) in 31.0 ml water and add 12.5 ml conc. acetic acid. Stir the reaction mixture overnight for 15 h, then concentrate the mixture to dryness under reduced pressure in a Büchi Rotavapor or equivalent rotary evaporator and dissolve the resulting white foaming solid in 19.0 ml anhydrous dimethylformamide (DMF).

2. Add 1.87 g potassium bicarbonate (18.7 mmol) and 2.25 ml 1-iodooctane (12.5 mmol) to the reaction mixture. Stir the reaction mixture for 15 h at room temperature, then dilute with 30.0 ml double distilled water (ddH$_2$O).

3. Extract the aqueous layer three times, each time with 70 ml ethyl acetate. Combine the ethyl acetate extracts, wash them with brine (saturated NaCl solution) and dry them over anhydrous sodium sulfate.

4. Evaporate the solvent under reduced pressure in a Büchi Rotavapor or equivalent rotary evaporator and purify the crude product by automated flash chromatography using a 40 g silica gel column, and a mixture of hexane and ethyl acetate, with a 20 ml/min flow rate. Initially, hold the gradient at 10% ethyl acetate for 15 min to elute the less polar compounds, and then increase the gradient to 30% ethyl acetate for 20 min to elute the more polar compounds. End the chromatography run once the fourth peak elutes. 5-benzyl 1-octyl (R)-2-hydroxypentanedioate will isolate as clear oil in the third peak with $R_T = 22$ min (~41% yield, ~0.900 g).

5. Synthesis of 5-benzyl 1-octyl (R)-2-hydroxypentanedioate can be confirmed by NMR spectroscopy. The spectrum is:

    ^{1}H NMR (500 MHz, Chloroform-*d*) δ 7.42–7.28 (m, 5H), 4.22 (ddd, *J* = 8.0, 5.4, 4.1 Hz, 1H), 4.18 (t, *J* = 6.8 Hz, 2H), 2.85 (tt, *J* = 5.3, 2.4 Hz, 1H), 2.63–2.39 (m, 2H), 2.27–2.12

(m, 1H), 1.98–1.87 (m, 1H), 1.69–1.60 (m, 2H), 1.38–1.21 (m, 12H), 0.88 (t, J=6.9 Hz, 3H). ^{13}C NMR (126 MHz, CDCl$_3$) δ 174.7, 172.9, 135.9, 128.6, 128.2, 128.2, 77.3, 69.4, 66.4, 66.1, 31.8, 29.7, 29.4, 29.1, 29.1, 28.5, 25.8, 22.6, 14.1.

6. Enantiomeric purity of the title compound can be measured at this step by reverse phase HPLC. The enantiomeric purity should be higher than 98%. The HPLC chromatogram of 5-benzyl 1-octyl (R)-2-hydroxypentanedioate (R_T=7.2 min) should be compared to a mixture of both R and S enantiomers (respectively R_T=7.2 min and 6.6 min).

3.1.3 Synthesis of (R)-4-hydroxy-5-(octyloxy)-5-oxopentanoic Acid

Schema for synthesis of (R)-4-hydroxy-5-(octyloxy)-5-oxopentanoic acid from 5-benzyl 1-octyl (R)-2-hydroxypentanedioate is shown in Fig. 2, bottom panel.

1. Add 300.0 mg 5-benzyl 1-octyl (R)-2-hydroxypentanedioate (0.856 mmol) to a three necked-round bottom flask equipped with a magnetic stirring bar, a nitrogen inlet adapter connected to a nitrogen/vacuum manifold, a rubber septum and a gas inlet adapter with a stopcock and a balloon filled with hydrogen. Evacuate and back-fill the flask with nitrogen 3 times, then add 20.0 ml anhydrous methanol, followed by 16.8 mg 10% (wt/wt) palladium on carbon while keeping the system under nitrogen atmosphere. Evacuate and back-fill the flask with hydrogen.

2. Stir the reaction for 1.5 h, then evacuate and back-fill with nitrogen.

3. Pour a celite pad (using a slurry of celite in ethyl acetate) on a glass Buchner-type filtration funnel with sintered disc, and connection for vacuum. Filter the mixture through this celite pad. Collect the filtrate.

4. Evaporate the solvent, and purify the crude material by automated flash chromatography, using a 16 g silica gel column with a mixture of ethyl acetate in hexanes with an 8 ml/min flow rate. Run the gradient from 10 to 30% ethyl acetate over 10 min, then hold at 30% for 7 min and increase to 50% ethyl acetate over the next 15 min, then to 100% ethyl acetate over the final 15 min of the chromatography run.

5. (R)-4-hydroxy-5-(octyloxy)-5-oxopentanoic acid (octyl-R-2-hydroxyglutarate, octyl-R2HG) is not UV active. It can be visualized by TLC with cerium ammonium molybdate stain Rf=0.13 and will isolate as colorless solid (~45% yield, ~100 mg) (*see* **Notes 2–4**). The specific optical rotation is $[\alpha]_D^{23}$ = +15° (c=0.28, CH$_2$Cl$_2$).

6. Synthesis of octyl-R2HG can be confirmed by NMR spectroscopy. The spectrum is:

¹H NMR (500 MHz, Chloroform-*d*) δ 4.24 (dd, *J*=8.0, 4.2 Hz, 1H), 4.19 (t, *J*=6.8 Hz, 2H), 2.65–2.45 (m, 2H), 2.19 (dddd, *J*=14.2, 8.3, 7.1, 4.2 Hz, 1H), 1.95 (dtd, *J*=14.2, 8.1, 6.1 Hz, 1H), 1.72–1.61 (m, 2H), 1.40–1.08 (m, 10H), 0.88 (t, *J*=6.9 Hz, 3H). ¹³C NMR (126 MHz, CDCl₃) δ 178.5, 174.7, 69.3, 66.2, 31.7, 29.4, 29.1 (2C), 29.0, 28.5, 25.8, 22.6, 14.1.

Calculated for $[M-H]^- = 259.1551$, found $ESI^- = 259.1546$, $\Delta = 2.0$ ppm.

3.2 Application of Octyl-R-2-hydroxyglutarate or Octyl-L-2-hydroxyglutarate to Inhibit Histone Demethylation in Mammalian Cells

The efficiency of inhibition of histone demethylation upon cellular exposure to octyl-R2HG or octyl-L2HG will vary according to the α-ketoglutarate-dependent histone methyltransferase being targeted, the concentration and length of time of exposure to octyl-R2HG or octyl-L2HG, as well as the cell type of interest (*see* **Notes 4** and **5**). Here, we describe strategies for inhibiting histone demethylation by Jumonji-domain containing demethylases, and monitoring H3 K79me2 levels in K-562 cells as an example (Fig. 3).

1. Seed four 60 mm cell culture plates with 1×10^6 cells in 3 ml media (e.g., for K-562 cells, complete IMDM, 10% FBS). Incubate the cells overnight at 37 °C with 5% CO₂ (*see* **Note 6**).

2. Dissolve octyl-L2HG or octyl-R2HG in PBS or media to final concentration of 10 mM (*see* **Note 6**).

3. For attachment-dependent cells, remove the media by aspiration, and add fresh media containing or lacking (e.g., 0, 1, 5, 10 mM) octyl-R2HG or octyl-L2HG to each plate. For attachment-independent cells, transfer cells to 15 ml conical tube, pellet cells by centrifugation at $300 \times g$ for 5 min, then

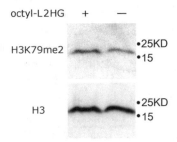

Fig. 3 Inhibition of histone demethylation by L2HG. H3K79me2 levels increased 1.7-fold in K-562 cells in the presence versus the absence of octyl-L2HG. 5×10^5 cell equivalents of whole cell extracts from K-562 cells that had been treated with 0 or 10 mM octyl-L2HG for 4 h were analyzed by immunoblotting with anti-H3 K79me2 antibodies (*top panel*), then stripped and reprobed with anti-H3 antibodies (*bottom panel*) as described in Sect. 3.4

remove media from the cell pellet by aspiration. Suspend the cell pellet in fresh media containing octyl-R2HG or octyl-L2HG as above and transfer to 60 mm cell culture plates.

4. Incubate the cells for 6 h at 37 °C with 5 % CO_2 prior to analyses as outlined in Sects. 3.3 or 3.4 (*see* **Note 4**).

3.3 Protein Extraction from Mammalian Cells

1. For attachment-dependent cells, remove media by aspiration, wash 1× with 3 ml PBS, then remove PBS. Add 0.3 ml Trypsin–EDTA and incubate for ~2 min to detach cells from plate. Add 3 ml fresh media (containing FBS) to plate to inactivate Trypsin and transfer cells suspended in media to a 15 ml conical tube. For attachment-independent cells (e.g., K-562), transfer all cells suspended in media directly to a 15 ml conical tube.

2. Pellet cells by centrifugation at $300 \times g$ for 5 min, then remove media from the cell pellet by aspiration. Suspend the cell pellet in 5 ml PBS at room temperature. Remove a 10 μl aliquot for counting cells on a hemocytometer (*see* **Note 7**).

3. Pellet cells by centrifugation at $300 \times g$ for 5 min, then remove PBS from the cell pellet by aspiration.

4. Make a stock solution of Extraction Buffer containing PMSF by adding 0.5 μl 0.2 M PMSF per 100 μl Extraction Buffer and store on ice until use. Add 100 μl Extraction Buffer containing PMSF per 1×10^6 cells, and suspend the cell pellets by pipetting up and down briefly.

5. Incubate the suspended cells on ice for 10 min.

6. Sonicate the samples (e.g., when using a microtip on a Branson Sonifier 450 sonicator, set to 20 % output power, constant duty cycle, and conduct 3–5 replicates of 30 s. of sonication, followed by 30 s. on ice (*see* **Note 8**)). Wash microtip with ethanol, then ddH_2O prior to processing each sample.

7. Transfer the sonicated sample to a microfuge tube and subject sample to centrifugation in a microcentrifuge at ~$14,000 \times g$ for 15 min. at 4 °C. Transfer the supernatant to a fresh tube and use immediately or store sample at −80 °C (*see* **Note 9**).

3.4 Monitoring Histone Methylation by Immunoblotting

Upon inhibition of Jumonji domain-containing histone demethylases by R2HG or L2HG, the levels of histone methylation will increase in treated relative to untreated cells. The impact of R2HG or L2HG on histone methylation can be readily monitored by immunoblotting, as outlined below for H3 K79me2 (Sects. 3.4.1–3.4.3; Fig. 3).

3.4.1 Electrophoresis and Protein Transfer

1. Assemble an electrophoresis apparatus (e.g., for Bio-Rad Mini-Protean Electrophoresis Tetra Cell System or equivalent) as per manufacturers' instructions.

2. For analysis of histones, prepare a 15% acrylamide running gel (15% acrylamide, 370 mM Tris–HCl, pH 8.8, 0.1% SDS, 0.075% APS, 0.075% TEMED). Mix acrylamide, Tris–HCl, SDS and water together, then add APS and TEMED last, mix, and pour gel immediately thereafter (*see* **Note 10**).

3. Add a thin layer of butanol on top of the 15% running gel to achieve an even transition between the stacking and running gels, and allow the gel to polymerize.

4. Once polymerized pour off butanol, rinse gel with ddH$_2$O, and insert well combs into apparatus.

5. Prepare 4% acrylamide stacking gel (4% acrylamide, 130 mM Tris–HCl pH6.8, 0.1% SDS, 0.1% APS and 0.1% TEMED). Mix as in **step 2** and immediately pour stacking gel on top of running gel. Ensure no bubbles are trapped in the gel and that the comb is level.

6. Once gels have polymerized, remove well combs and rinse wells with SDS-PAGE Running Buffer by pipetting, and complete assembly of electrophoresis apparatus as per manufacturer' instructions.

7. Mix 5×10^5 cell equivalents of protein extracts from Sect. 3.3 with ¼ volume 4× Loading Buffer containing β-mercaptoethanol. Boil samples for 5 min at 100 °C prior to loading gel.

8. Load gel with a Protein Molecular Weight Ladder and samples. Separate proteins by electrophoresis (20 V/cm) for ~2 h, stopping electrophoresis when the loading dye is 1–2 cm from the bottom of the gel.

9. Disassemble electrophoresis apparatus and place gel on top of two sheets of Whatman paper that have been pre-wetted in Transfer Buffer. Pre-wet a PVDF membrane in methanol, then Transfer Buffer. Place PVDF membrane on top of gel, then place two sheets of pre-wetted Whatman paper on top of membrane. Remove bubbles after adding each layer to the stack by rolling a pipette across the top of the stack. Assemble the transfer apparatus according to manufacturer's instructions, with the membrane facing the positive, and the gel facing the negative, pole of the apparatus. Transfer proteins to the membrane by electrophoresis (~100 V for one hour) according to manufacturers' instructions.

10. Disassemble the transfer apparatus and place membrane onto a dry piece of Whatman paper. Allow the membrane to air-dry, with protein side facing up to bind proteins covalently to the membrane.

3.4.2 Immunoblotting

1. Incubate the membrane, with protein side facing up, in Blocking Buffer overnight at 4 °C (*see* **Note 11**).

2. Dilute the primary antibody (1:2000 for rabbit polyclonal anti-histone H3K79me2 antibodies, Upstate #07–366) in 4 ml fresh Blocking Buffer (*see* **Note 12**).

3. Remove the Blocking Buffer from the membrane. Add the diluted primary antibody to the membrane, and rock the membrane gently for 1 h at room temperature (*see* **Note 13**).

4. Wash the membrane three times in 5 ml PBST for 5 min. each at room temperature with gentle rocking. Remove last wash from membrane.

5. Dilute the secondary antibody (1:10,000 for donkey polyclonal anti-Rabbit IgG, GE Healthcare #NA934) in 5 ml Blocking Buffer, and apply to the membrane (*see* **Notes 12** and **13**). Gently rock the membrane for 1 h at room temperature.

6. Wash the membrane three times as in **step 4**.

7. Wash the membrane once in 5 ml PBS for 5 min., then remove PBS.

8. Image and quantify the target protein using the technique compatible with the secondary antibody (e.g., for chemiluminescence-based detection Luminata Crescendo Western HRP Substrate #WBLUR01500 for HRP-conjugated secondary antibodies) as per manufacturer's instructions.

9. Image membrane and collect quantification data from bands on membrane using a Chemimager and associated software (e.g., Bio-Rad ChemiDoc XRS+ or equivalent) as per manufacturer's instructions.

10. Strip membrane as described in Sect. 3.4.3, then re-probe with anti-histone H3 antibodies (1:5,000 for polyclonal anti-histone H3 antibodies, Abcam #1791) plus an appropriate secondary antibody (1:10,000 for donkey polyclonal anti-Rabbit IgG, GE Healthcare #NA934) and analyze as outlined above as a control for sample loading (*see* **Notes 12** and **13**).

11. Calculate the relative change in histone methylation levels in the absence versus the presence of oncometabolite as follows: $(H3K79me2/H3)_{treatment}/(H3K72me2/H3)_{no\ treatment}$, where treatment = incubation of cells with metabolite, L2HG or R2HG.

3.4.3 Stripping Membranes

1. To strip membrane for re-probing, wash the membrane three times in 5–10 ml 0.2 M NaOH for 10 min. each at room temperature.

2. Wash the membrane three times in 5–10 ml PBST for 5 min. each at room temperature.

3. Wash the membrane once in 5–10 ml PBS for 5 min. at room temperature.

4. Confirm that the antibodies have been removed by re-imaging blot as in **step 9** of Sect. 3.4.2. Repeat **steps 1–3** if residual signal is observed upon re-imaging.

---

4   Notes

1. For the synthesis of octyl-L-2-hydroxyglutarate instead of octyl-R-2-hydroxyglutarate, L-glutamic acid should be used instead of D-glutamic acid during the first step in synthesis as outlined in Sect. 3.1.1 (*see* Fig. 2). Briefly, (L)-2-amino-5-(benzyloxy)-5-oxopentanoic acid is synthesized from benzyl alcohol and L-glutamic acid; 5-benzyl 1-octyl (L)-2-hydroxypentanedioate is synthesized from (L)-2-amino-5-(benzyloxy)-5-oxopentanoic acid; (L)-4-hydroxy-5-(octyloxy)-5-oxopentanoic acid is synthesized from 5-benzyl 1-octyl (L)-2-hydroxypentanedioate.

2. Synthesis of octyl-L2HG can be confirmed by NMR spectroscopy and octyl-L2HG will have the same spectrum as octyl-R2HG (*see* Sect. 3.1.3).

3. Replacing methanol with the less polar ethyl acetate may reduce the rate of the reaction and afford higher yields.

4. Isolated octyl-R2HG and octyl-L2HG should be stored at 4 °C under desiccation.

5. The working concentration of octyl-L2HG or octyl-R2HG as well as incubation times should be optimized empirically for cell lines and chromatin-modifying enzymes of interest. In cells expressing IDH mutants, R2HG is elevated, and can accumulate to >10 mM [24, 26, 27]. Incubation of glioblastoma cells that express wild-type IDH1/2 in lower levels of R2HG can enhance cell migration and promote colony formation in soft agar assays [49]. However, prolonged exposure to R2HG can also inhibit cell growth and lead to cell death for certain cell types [49, 50].

6. Upon cellular entry, octyl-R2HG and octyl-L2HG will be hydrolyzed by cellular esterases, releasing R2HG or L2HG.

7. Resuspended octyl-L2HG or octyl-R2HG may be stored at −20 °C for limited periods prior to use.

8. To count cells, add 10 μl of cells to 90 μl of 0.4% (w/v) Trypan Blue and apply mixture to a hemocytometer. Count the four large squares, ensuring that at least 50 cells were counted, and divide by four. Multiple by 100,000 to convert to cells/ml.

9. The cell mixture may become viscous after incubation on ice, but will lose viscosity after sonication. Use the minimum number of sonication cycles necessary to reduce viscosity. For additional details on immunoblotting, *see* [51–54].

10. Histone extracts can alternatively be prepared by high salt or acid extraction [55].

11. The percent acrylamide in the running gel and electrophoresis conditions will vary, depending on the size and electrophoretic mobility behavior of the targeted protein.

12. Incubation in Blocking Buffer can alternatively be conducted at room temperature for 1 h.

13. Dilute antibodies as per manufacturer's instructions prior to use. Optimal concentrations and incubation conditions required to enrich for signal and to reduce nonspecific background should be determined empirically.

14. Keep the membrane wet to prevent the antibodies from becoming irreversibly bound to the membrane.

Acknowledgments

This work was supported by the W.M. Keck Foundation (A.L.K.), Purdue University Center for Cancer Research (http://www.cancerresearch.purdue.edu) Innovative Pilot and Shared Resource Grants (A.L.K.), and a Bird Stair Fellowship (H.B.). This research was also supported by the National Cancer Institute (http://www.cancer.gov) [CCSG CA23168] for data acquired in the Purdue Computational and Medicinal Chemistry Resource.

References

1. Jeschke J, Collignon E, Fuks F (2016) Portraits of TET-mediated DNA hydroxymethylation in cancer. Curr Opin Genet Dev 36:16–26. doi:10.1016/j.gde.2016.01.004

2. Tan L, Shi YG (2012) Tet family proteins and 5-hydroxymethylcytosine in development and disease. Development 139:1895–1902. doi:10.1242/dev.070771

3. Ko M, An J, Rao A (2015) DNA methylation and hydroxymethylation in hematologic differentiation and transformation. Curr Opin Cell Biol 37:91–101. doi:10.1016/j.ceb.2015.10.009

4. Caren H, Pollard SM, Beck S (2013) The good, the bad and the ugly: epigenetic mechanisms in glioblastoma. Mol Asp Med 34:849–862. doi:10.1016/j.mam.2012.06.007

5. Rose NR, Woon EC, Tumber A et al (2012) Plant growth regulator daminozide is a selective inhibitor of human KDM2/7 histone demethylases. J Med Chem 55:6639–6643. doi:10.1021/jm300677j

6. Chowdhury R, Yeoh KK, Tian YM et al (2011) The oncometabolite 2-hydroxyglutarate inhibits histone lysine demethylases. EMBO Rep 12:463–469. doi:10.1038/embor.2011.43

7. Lu C, Ward PS, Kapoor GS et al (2012) IDH mutation impairs histone demethylation and results in a block to cell differentiation. Nature 483:474–478. doi:10.1038/nature10860

8. Xu W, Yang H, Liu Y et al (2011) Oncometabolite 2-hydroxyglutarate is a competitive inhibitor of alpha-ketoglutarate-dependent dioxygenases. Cancer Cell 19:17–30. doi:10.1016/j.ccr.2010.12.014

9. Zhang Y, Jurkowska R, Soeroes S et al (2010) Chromatin methylation activity of Dnmt3a and Dnmt3a/3L is guided by interaction of

the ADD domain with the histone H3 tail. Nucleic Acids Res 38:4246–4253. doi:10.1093/nar/gkq147

10. Li BZ, Huang Z, Cui QY et al (2011) Histone tails regulate DNA methylation by allosterically activating de novo methyltransferase. Cell Res 21:1172–1181. doi:10.1038/cr.2011.92

11. Guo X, Wang L, Li J et al (2015) Structural insight into autoinhibition and histone H3-induced activation of DNMT3A. Nature 517:640–644. doi:10.1038/nature13899

12. Valinluck V, Sowers LC (2007) Endogenous cytosine damage products alter the site selectivity of human DNA maintenance methyltransferase DNMT1. Cancer Res 67:946–950. doi:10.1158/0008-5472. CAN-06-3123

13. Hashimoto H, Liu Y, Upadhyay AK et al (2012) Recognition and potential mechanisms for replication and erasure of cytosine hydroxymethylation. Nucleic Acids Res 40:4841–4849. doi:10.1093/nar/gks155

14. He YF, Li BZ, Li Z et al (2011) Tet-mediated formation of 5-carboxylcytosine and its excision by TDG in mammalian DNA. Science 333:1303–1307. doi:10.1126/science.1210944

15. Ito S, Shen L, Dai Q et al (2011) Tet proteins can convert 5-methylcytosine to 5-formylcytosine and 5-carboxylcytosine. Science 333:1300–1303. doi:10.1126/science.1210597

16. Maiti A, Drohat AC (2011) Thymine DNA glycosylase can rapidly excise 5-formylcytosine and 5-carboxylcytosine: potential implications for active demethylation of CpG sites. J Biol Chem 286:35334–35338. doi:10.1074/jbc. C111.284620

17. Zhang L, Lu X, Lu J et al (2012) Thymine DNA glycosylase specifically recognizes 5-carboxylcytosine-modified DNA. Nat Chem Biol 8:328–330. doi:10.1038/nchembio.914

18. Guo JU, Su Y, Zhong C et al (2011) Hydroxylation of 5-methylcytosine by TET1 promotes active DNA demethylation in the adult brain. Cell 145:423–434. doi:10.1016/j. cell.2011.03.022

19. Lindahl G, Lindstedt G, Lindstedt S (1967) Metabolism of 2-amino-5-hydroxyadipic acid in the rat. Arch Biochem Biophys 119:347–352

20. Chalmers RA, Lawson AM, Watts RW et al (1980) D-2-hydroxyglutaric aciduria: case report and biochemical studies. J Inherit Metab Dis 3:11–15

21. Rzem R, Veiga-da-Cunha M, Noel G et al (2004) A gene encoding a putative FAD-dependent L-2-hydroxyglutarate dehydrogenase is mutated in L-2-hydroxyglutaric aciduria. Proc Natl Acad Sci U S A 101:16849–16854. doi:10.1073/pnas.0404840101

22. Achouri Y, Noel G, Vertommen D et al (2004) Identification of a dehydrogenase acting on D-2-hydroxyglutarate. Biochem J 381(Pt 1):35–42. doi:10.1042/BJ20031933

23. Struys EA, Salomons GS, Achouri Y et al (2005) Mutations in the D-2-hydroxyglutarate dehydrogenase gene cause D-2-hydroxyglutaric aciduria. Am J Hum Genet 76:358–360. doi:10.1086/427890

24. Dang L, White DW, Gross S et al (2009) Cancer-associated IDH1 mutations produce 2-hydroxyglutarate. Nature 462:739–744. doi:10.1038/nature08617

25. Losman JA, Kaelin WG Jr (2013) What a difference a hydroxyl makes: mutant IDH, (R)-2-hydroxyglutarate, and cancer. Genes Dev 27:836–852. doi:10.1101/gad.217406.113

26. Gross S, Cairns RA, Minden MD et al (2010) Cancer-associated metabolite 2-hydroxyglutarate accumulates in acute myelogenous leukemia with isocitrate dehydrogenase 1 and 2 mutations. J Exp Med 207:339–344. doi:10.1084/jem.20092506

27. Ward PS, Patel J, Wise DR et al (2010) The common feature of leukemia-associated IDH1 and IDH2 mutations is a neomorphic enzyme activity converting alpha-ketoglutarate to 2-hydroxyglutarate. Cancer Cell 17:225–234. doi:10.1016/j.ccr.2010.01.020

28. Borger DR, Tanabe KK, Fan KC et al (2012) Frequent mutation of isocitrate dehydrogenase (IDH)1 and IDH2 in cholangiocarcinoma identified through broad-based tumor genotyping. Oncologist 17:72–79. doi:10.1634/theoncologist.2011-0386

29. Cairns RA, Iqbal J, Lemonnier F et al (2012) IDH2 mutations are frequent in angioimmunoblastic T-cell lymphoma. Blood 119:1901–1903. doi:10.1182/blood-2011-11-391748

30. Yan H, Parsons DW, Jin G et al (2009) IDH1 and IDH2 mutations in gliomas. N Engl J Med 360:765–773. doi:10.1056/NEJMoa0808710

31. Mardis ER, Ding L, Dooling DJ et al (2009) Recurring mutations found by sequencing an acute myeloid leukemia genome. N Engl J Med 361:1058–1066. doi:10.1056/NEJMoa0903840

32. Parsons DW, Jones S, Zhang X et al (2008) An integrated genomic analysis of human glioblastoma multiforme. Science 321:1807–1812. doi:10.1126/science.1164382

33. Jin G, Reitman ZJ, Duncan CG et al (2013) Disruption of wild-type IDH1 suppresses

D-2-hydroxyglutarate production in IDH1-mutated gliomas. Cancer Res 73:496–501. doi:10.1158/0008-5472.CAN-12-2852

34. Rendina AR, Pietrak B, Smallwood A et al (2013) Mutant IDH1 enhances the production of 2-hydroxyglutarate due to its kinetic mechanism. Biochemistry 52:4563–4577. doi:10.1021/bi400514k

35. Ward PS, Lu C, Cross JR et al (2013) The potential for isocitrate dehydrogenase mutations to produce 2-hydroxyglutarate depends on allele specificity and subcellular compartmentalization. J Biol Chem 288:3804–3815. doi:10.1074/jbc.M112.435495

36. Losman JA, Looper RE, Koivunen P et al (2013) (R)-2-hydroxyglutarate is sufficient to promote leukemogenesis and its effects are reversible. Science 339:1621–1625. doi:10.1126/science.1231677

37. Shim EH, Livi CB, Rakheja D et al (2014) L-2-Hydroxyglutarate: an epigenetic modifier and putative oncometabolite in renal cancer. Cancer Discov 4:1290–1298. doi:10.1158/2159-8290.CD-13-0696

38. Rzem R, Vincent MF, Van Schaftingen E et al (2007) L-2-hydroxyglutaric aciduria, a defect of metabolite repair. J Inherit Metab Dis 30:681–689. doi:10.1007/s10545-007-0487-0

39. Schatz L, Segal HL (1969) Reduction of alpha-ketoglutarate by homogeneous lactic dehydrogenase X of testicular tissue. J Biol Chem 244:4393–4397

40. Oldham WM, Clish CB, Yang Y et al (2015) Hypoxia-mediated increases in l-2-hydroxyglutarate coordinate the metabolic response to reductive stress. Cell Metab 22:291–303. doi:10.1016/j.cmet.2015.06.021

41. Intlekofer AM, Dematteo RG, Venneti S et al (2015) Hypoxia induces production of L-2-hydroxyglutarate. Cell Metab 22:304–311. doi:10.1016/j.cmet.2015.06.023

42. Koivunen P, Lee S, Duncan CG et al (2012) Transformation by the (R)-enantiomer of 2-hydroxyglutarate linked to EGLN activation. Nature 483:484–488. doi:10.1038/nature10898

43. Rzem R, Van Schaftingen E, Veiga-da-Cunha M (2006) The gene mutated in l-2-hydroxyglutaric aciduria encodes l-2-hydroxyglutarate dehydrogenase. Biochimie 88:113–116. doi:10.1016/j.biochi.2005.06.005

44. Shim EH, Sudarshan S (2015) Another small molecule in the oncometabolite mix: L-2-Hydroxyglutarate in kidney cancer. Oncoscience 2:483–486

45. Hirata M, Sasaki M, Cairns RA et al (2015) Mutant IDH is sufficient to initiate enchondromatosis in mice. Proc Natl Acad Sci U S A 112:2829–2834. doi:10.1073/pnas.1424400112

46. Reitman ZJ, Duncan CG, Poteet E et al (2014) Cancer-associated isocitrate dehydrogenase 1 (IDH1) R132H mutation and d-2-hydroxyglutarate stimulate glutamine metabolism under hypoxia. J Biol Chem 289:23318–23328. doi:10.1074/jbc.M114.575183

47. Saha SK, Parachoniak CA, Ghanta KS et al (2014) Mutant IDH inhibits HNF-4alpha to block hepatocyte differentiation and promote biliary cancer. Nature 513:110–114. doi:10.1038/nature13441

48. Huang J, Chin R, Diep S et al. (2015) Compositions and methods for treating aging and age-related diseases and symptoms. U.S. Patent PCT/US2015/015304

49. Pusch S, Schweizer L, Beck AC et al (2014) D-2-Hydroxyglutarate producing neo-enzymatic activity inversely correlates with frequency of the type of isocitrate dehydrogenase 1 mutations found in glioma. Acta Neuropathol Commun 2:19. doi:10.1186/2051-5960-2-19

50. Balduf H, Kirchmaier AL (Unpublished)

51. Hnasko TS, Hnasko RM (2015) The western blot. Methods Mol Biol 1318:87–96. doi:10.1007/978-1-4939-2742-5_9

52. Burnette WN (1981) "Western blotting": electrophoretic transfer of proteins from sodium dodecyl sulfate--polyacrylamide gels to unmodified nitrocellulose and radiographic detection with antibody and radioiodinated protein A. Anal Biochem 112:195–203

53. Burnette WN (2009) Western blotting: remembrance of past things. Methods Mol Biol 536:5–8. doi:10.1007/978-1-59745-542-8_2

54. Mahmood T, Yang PC (2012) Western blot: technique, theory, and trouble shooting. N Am J Med Sci 4:429–434. doi:10.4103/1947-2714.100998

55. Shechter D, Dormann HL, Allis CD et al (2007) Extraction, purification and analysis of histones. Nat Protoc 2:1445–1457. doi:10.1038/nprot.2007.202

Chapter 6

High-Throughput Screening of Small Molecule Transcriptional Regulators in Embryonic Stem Cells Using qRT-PCR

Emily C. Dykhuizen, Leigh C. Carmody, and Nicola J. Tolliday

Abstract

While quantitative real-time reverse transcription polymerase chain reaction (qRT-PCR) is a standard tool for many laboratories studying gene regulation, it is not commonly used for small molecule screening. More commonly, high throughput screens (HTSs) designed to detect transcriptional changes use a gene reporter, such as green fluorescent protein (GFP), β-galactosidase, or luciferase. The downsides of this approach include the genetic manipulation required to make reporter lines, the artifacts introduced by this indirect measurement, and the limited number of genes that can be monitored. Here we describe a method for using qRT-PCR to assay the regulation of multiple genes in a 384-well format. We envision this technology being utilized in three main scenarios: screening against cell lines that are not amenable to genetic manipulation (such as lines derived from patients), screening for transcriptional regulators without well-defined functions, or as a secondary screen validating results obtained using a traditional reporter cell line or biochemical readout. Additionally, we provide useful guidelines and protocols for culturing and plating mouse embryonic stem (ES) cells for high throughput screening. While embryonic stem cells are of great interest for regenerative medicine and are a useful tool for studying the epigenetic regulation of cell identity, they are difficult to culture and require extra care and consideration. We provide a method for culturing and plating mouse ES cells in 384-well format.

Key words High-throughput screening, Embryonic stem cells, Epigenetics, qRT-PCR, Transcriptional assay, Real-time PCR

1 Small Molecule-Mediated Regulation of Transcription

The regulation of transcription is critical for many cellular processes, including differentiation, metabolism, and cell signaling. Many hundreds of proteins are involved in regulating transcription, from well-defined transcription factors to hundreds of less well-defined epigenetic regulators. These can include histone/DNA modifiers, micro and noncoding RNA, and chromatin readers and remodelers. While high throughput screening is commonly used to identify small molecules that inhibit these classes of transcriptional regulators, screens are typically performed on purified

Barbara Stefanska and David J. MacEwan (eds.), *Epigenetics and Gene Expression in Cancer, Inflammatory and Immune Diseases*, Methods in Pharmacology and Toxicology, DOI 10.1007/978-1-4939-6743-8_6, © Springer Science+Business Media LLC 2017

proteins and enzymes using biochemical readouts. While biochemical screens are very successful at identifying compounds that act in vitro, they often are not functional in a cell-based system. As such, there is a push to return to the so-called "phenotypic screens" as opposed to "target-based screens" [1]. If transcriptional regulation of a particular gene is the desired phenotype for a therapeutically useful small molecule, developing cell-based screen with a transcriptional readout should be the ultimate goal. As such, qRT-PCR provides the most direct readout of transcription and is less likely to be plagued with the artifacts commonly observed with fluorescence or enzymatic reporters [2, 3].

Traditional methods for screening for a transcriptional regulator utilize a fluorescent or enzymatic reporter protein. In addition to introducing artifacts, the utility of the reporter gene strategy is limited by the available mechanistic knowledge of transcriptional regulation. For example, genomic looping is important in the regulation of genes by enhancer elements hundreds of kilobases away [4]. Looping is particularly important in embryonic stem cells where long-range interactions are critical for the regulation of pluripotency genes [5]. This type of long-range regulation makes it very difficult to design a transgenic or vector-based reporter construct with the necessary elements for transcriptional regulation. While a small genetic region surrounding the transcription start site may be sufficient to screen for small molecules that disrupt transcription factor activity, it is not sufficient to screen for small molecules that target epigenetic regulators that act from a distance, such as chromatin remodelers [6].

For our studies, we were interested in developing inhibitors of the function of the mammalian SWI/SNF or BAF chromatin remodeling complex. [7] It is required for pluripotency in embryonic stem cells [8], development and differentiation [9], and is frequently mutated in cancer [10]. Although the BAF complex has known in vitro nucleosome remodeling and ATPase activity, it also has transcriptional effects separate from its nucleosome remodeling/ATPase activity, making a biochemical assay of ATPase activity potentially not reflective of in vivo function [11]. In addition, while only four subunits are required for its enzymatic ATPase activity [12], the other 8–10 subunits are required for in vivo activity, indicating other potential modes of inhibition that would be missed using a strictly biochemical assay. Lastly, as is that case for the majority of proteins in the nucleus, subunits of chromatin remodeling complexes exist and act together as a unit that is difficult to reconstitute in vitro, making a biochemical assay technically challenging. Because of all these factors, a cell-based assay of transcriptional function was the best option for screening for inhibitors of this complex transcriptional regulator.

2 Designing the qRT-PCR Assay

2.1 Selection of a Reporter Gene

If the screen is designed to detect the regulation of a therapeutic target in a relevant disease model, the gene of interest will already be known. However, if screening for inhibitors of a particular transcriptional regulator, it is important to carefully identify and validate a robust target in the cell type of choice. For example, we used ChIP-seq and microarray data from a conditional *Brg1* knockout ES cell line to identify transcriptional targets of the BAF chromatin remodeling complex in ES cells [13]. We chose *Bmi1* as our primary reporter of BAF activity for three main reasons: (1) Detecting an increase in gene expression is less prone to false positives than detecting a decrease in gene expression (2) *Bmi1* induction was one of the most robust targets, with a 10-fold increase of expression upon *Brg1* knockdown. (3) *Bmi1* is a particularly interesting target due to its essential role in the maintenance and self-renewal of hematopoietic and neural stem cells, as well as its role as an oncogene [14]. Thus, although our primary focus was to identify inhibitors of chromatin remodeling, compounds that regulate the expression of *Bmi1* independent of the BAF complex are also of interest. In fact, since our screen, small molecules that downregulate *Bmi1* transcript levels have been shown to prevent cancer in a mouse model for colorectal cancer [15]. As the saying goes, "you get what you screen for," so selecting an interesting reporter gene will guarantee that you are able to identify compounds that are of interest to a wider audience.

2.2 Validation of the Reporter Gene

Using the cell type of choice, develop a knockdown system using RNAi to validate the target. The cDNA from these cells can also serve as a positive control in the screen if no known small molecule regulator already exists. We validated *Bmi1* as a target of the BAF complex in ES cells using a standard SYBR qRT-PCR protocol (TRIzol® RNA isolation followed by cDNA synthesis using Life Technologies SuperScript® III First Strand Synthesis System followed by qPCR using Roche SYBR mastermix) and observed a tenfold increase of *Bmi1* expression upon *Brg1* knockdown in an ES cell line. We utilized the cDNA from this preparation as a positive control for the HTS, as well as to verify results from the Cells-to-C_T™ assay.

3 Optimizing the Cells-to-C_T™ qRT-PCR Assay

Optimization is key for the success of any high throughput screen. For additional in-depth protocols for implementation of high-throughput RT-PCR for small-molecule screening assays using other cell types, including data analysis, see the protocols described by Bittker [16]. We chose Taqman® probes (or any sequence specific fluorophore–quencher pair) as our qPCR readout as opposed to SYBR (a nonspecific intercalator that can be used with any PCR primer set). Although SYBR primers are cheaper and easier to optimize, a screen using SYBR requires duplicate plates in order to normalize gene expression using a housekeeping gene. In contrast, hydrolysable Taqman® probes with different fluorophores can be analyzed simultaneously in the same reaction, as most real time machines are easily able to detect at least two compatible dyes, VIC and FAM. The screen is simpler and more robust using Taqman® probes, but requires additional optimization up front.

3.1 Determine Timeline

Cells should be plated for 24 h before compound treatment. The duration of compound treatment will depend on the desired readout. As opposed to a reporter, qRT-PCR allows for the direct detection of transcriptional changes without requiring time to allow for translation and accumulation of the reporter. Thus, the assay can potentially detect transcriptional changes in the matter of minutes. However, since epigenetic regulators may take hours or even days to alter the chromatin landscape in such a way to change transcription, many screens allow for 24–48 h of compound treatment. If treating for more than 48 h, compound stability may start to be concern, and incubations over 72 h should be redosed.

3.2 Confirming Robust Readout Using HTS System

First confirm that using Ambion®'s Cells-to-C_T™ system with Applied Biosystem's Taqman® probes can replicate the transcriptional changes observed using your qRT-PCR methods (Fig. 1a). If the effect can be replicated, continue using the Cells-to-C_T™ system to optimize the following individual assay parameters for successful assay execution in 384-well format.

3.3 Selection of the Housekeeping Gene and Multiplexing

A serious concern is the selection of an appropriate housekeeping gene, as it is always possible that inhibiting a transcriptional regulator can affect mRNA levels of the so-called housekeeping genes. We surveyed a panel of housekeeping genes to confirm similar expression levels upon *Brg1* knockdown (Fig. 1b). We found that *Gapdh*, *Actin*, and *Hsp90* all have similar expression levels in response to *Brg1* knockdown. Based on this data, we selected both the actin and *Gapdh* Taqman® probes to compare for multiplexing *Bmi1* with a housekeeping gene. When we ran concentration curves with *Bmi1* multiplexed with *Actin* or *Gapdh*, we found that *Actin* worked better for multiplexing (Fig. 1c), as the primers for *Gapdh* lost efficiency at high concentrations of cDNA.

3.4 Primer Efficiency

Primer efficiency is critical for proper hit selection. To simplify the analysis of the screen data, we performed calculations based on the $2^{-\Delta\Delta CT}$ calculations described by Livak and Schmittgen [17]. To use this calculation, it is critical that primer efficiencies are the same

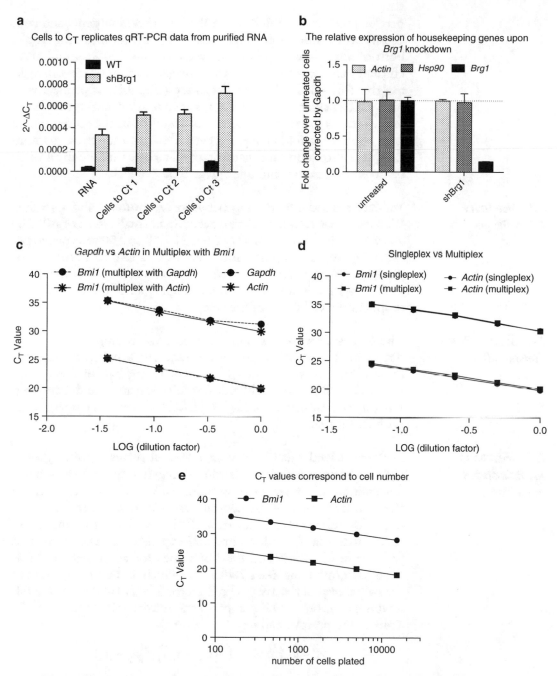

Fig. 1 Several parameters should be optimized before proceeding with a Taqman®-based qRT-PCR screen, as illustrated by the following figures. (**a**) Verify that biological data obtained with other qRT-PCR system is replicated using the Cells-to-C$_T$™ system in 384-well format, (**b**) Choose an appropriate housekeeping gene that is not altered in any way by the transcriptional regulator being screened. In this example, *Actin*, *Gapdh*, and *Hsp90* are all suitable housekeeping genes. (**c**) Screen several housekeeping gene primers to determine which multiplexes better with the target of interest. In this example, *Gapdh* loses efficiency at high cDNA concentrations and is not a suitable housekeeping gene primer set. (**d**) Determine that primers behave similarly in multiplex and in singleplex, and that the both primer sets have adequate, and most importantly, similar amplification efficiencies. (**e**) Verify that primer amplification is consistent over a range of plated cell numbers

between the gene of interest and the housekeeping gene, and consistent over a wide range of transcript concentrations. For example, both of our primer sets have between 97 and 100% amplification efficiency and are sensitive down to very low transcript levels, making this simplified calculation accurate (Fig. 1d). If primers with high efficiency are unavailable, a concentration curve that accurately reflects the range of C_T values observed in the screen can be used to derive a fold change or even absolute transcript quantitation. It is also important that primer efficiencies are identical when detected alone or in multiplex (Fig. 1d).

3.5 Determine Assay Range

Validate a direct relationship between cell number and C_T value. We found that ΔC_T provides an accurate normalization of *Bmi1* by *Actin* for cell numbers ranging from 15,000 to 150 cells plated per well (Fig. 1e). This optimization verifies an appropriate density for plating cells to prevent confluency, but also verifies that the Cells-to-C_T™ system is able to accurately amplify all of the desired transcripts in the cell range of the assay.

3.6 Taqman Probe Concentration

The biggest downside of qRT-PCR-based screening is the cost. By decreasing the concentration of the Taqman® probes, we were able to save on the cost of the qPCR step. Using half of the recommended amount gave us identical results as using the full amount, but this optimization should be performed for every new primer probe set tested.

3.7 Measuring the Robustness of the Assay

Perform several small screens in 384-well plates consisting of at least 24 positive control wells and 24 negative control wells. Then determine the coefficient of variation (CV), which is the ratio of the standard deviation of neutral controls to the mean. For any high throughput screen effort, a CV below 10% is required. We determined that CV values for *Bmi1* expression in DMSO-treated wells were 0.6–2.4% and the CV values for actin were 1–3.6%. Next, determine the Z-factor (or Z′), which is the true measure of the robustness of the assay. The Z-factor is calculated using the following equation, which compares the means and standard deviations of the positive and negative controls:

$$Z' - \text{factor} = 1 - \left(3\left(\sigma_p + \sigma_n\right)\right) / \left|\mu_p - \mu_n\right|$$

σ_p = std. dev. of the pos. controls, σ_p = std. dev. of the neg. controls
μ_p = mean of the pos. controls, μ_n = mean of the neg. controls

The Z-factor for the transcriptional assay was 0.9, making it an extremely robust assay (robust assays have Z′ ≥0.5). *See* Fig. 2 for an illustration of how this data should look plotted as individual compound-treated wells.

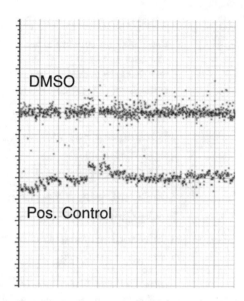

Fig. 2 An initial test screen consisting of several positive and negative controls should be run to determine the coefficient of variation (CV) and Z′ (comparison of standard deviation and means of the positive and negative controls. In this example of a very robust qRT-PCR screen (CV = 2% and Z′ = 0.9), each well is depicted as a point, illustrating the clear division between positive and negative controls

3.8 **Pilot Screen**

The pilot screen is critical for determining the feasibility of any assay. While preliminary data and optimization may look good, the decision to implement a costly screen with this many transfer steps will depend on the data from this small pilot. A pilot screen generally utilizes 500–2000 compounds screened in duplicate or triplicate. It typically consists of compounds with known bioactivity (including FDA-approved drugs), although it will ideally represent the composition of the final screening library. All plates need to include neutral controls (DMSO alone) and positive controls. At least 24 wells need to be DMSO controls in order to make accurate $-\Delta\Delta C_T$ calculations. As for positive controls, 8–12 wells is sufficient. The hit cutoff will be assay dependent. Using a hit cutoff of at least a 2.5-fold increase in *Bmi1* levels, 12 hits were identified from our pilot screen, giving a hit rate of 0.55%. This is in contrast to hit rates of 2% or more for luciferase screens, which mostly consists of artifacts.

4 Cell Culture

Media conditions for mouse ES cell culture:

High-glucose Dulbecco's modified Eagle's medium (DMEM; Invitrogen, Carlsbad, CA).

15 % fetal bovine serum (FBS; ES cell qualified; Applied Stem Cell.

note: Many commercial lots of FBS will be suitable for ES cell work; they just have not been qualified. We often request samples of multiple lots and test them for maintenance of pluripotency and buy large quantities of a suitable lot for our ES cell work.

100 μM 2-mercaptoethanol (Invitrogen).

1 % minimum essential medium (MEM) nonessential amino acids (Invitrogen).

1 mM Hepes (Invitrogen).

100 U/mL pen/strep (Invitrogen).

2 mM GlutaMAX™ (Invitrogen).

1 mM sodium pyruvate (Invitrogen).

1 U/mL LIF (Millipore).

note: LIF can be inexpensively obtained from the conditioned media of cos7 cells transfected with a LIF expressing construct. Harvest a large batch of media from confluent cos7 cells and test dilutions on ES cells. We find up to 1:5000 dilutions are often sufficient to support ES cell growth.

4.1 Making Feeder Free ES cell lines

Embryonic stem cells are traditionally very difficult to culture, making high throughput screening a challenge. When deriving mouse ES cells from blastocysts, they require culture on a layer of irradiated mouse embryonic fibroblasts plated on gelatin-coated plates. These feeder cells are costly, labor-intensive and cumbersome for screening. Most importantly, they confound transcriptional readouts. The first step for developing a line suitable for screening is to make the desired ES cell line feeder-free.

1. Derive or obtain a suitable ES cell line on MEF feeders.
2. Pretreat standard tissue culture treated plates for 30 min with 0.1 % gelatin in water (Millipore).
3. Aspirate gelatin
4. To make a feeder-free line, plate the ES cells at a high density (5 million cells on a 10 cm dish or 1.7 million cells for a 6 cm dish).
5. Split cells every 3 days at the same density onto gelatin-coated plates. The cells will initially look overgrown and differentiated, but by passage 4 or 5, the colonies will appear round and compact again (*see* Fig. 3 for an example of proper feeder free morphology).
6. After this point, the cells may need to be plated at a lower density for continued passage. The cells should be passaged at a density that allows 2–3 days of growth at which point the colonies are close but not quite touching. The exact density is cell line-dependent, but often between two and four million cells for a 10 cm dish.

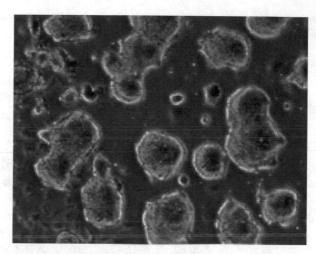

Fig. 3 Proper ES cell culture results in distinct, well-defined, round, three-dimensional colonies with edges close to each other, but not touching, after 2–3 days of growth

4.2 Plating Feeder Free ES Cells for HTS Efforts

1. Pretreat 384-well tissue culture plates with gelatin (20 μL/well) for at least 30 min at room temperature.

   Plates can be incubated with gelatin in advance and stored at room temperature for several days.

2. Remove gelatin by aspiration using a 12-channel aspiration wand.

   If an aspiration wand is not available, the plates can be spun upside-down in a centrifuge onto sterile paper towels at 50×g. The surface tension in 384-well plates can make it difficult to remove media easily so it is critical to use a robust method to remove all gelatin before plating cells.

3. Plate 5000 ES cells per well in a total volume of 50 μL ES media using a Thermo Multidrop™ Combi reagent dispenser.

   A reagent dispenser helps to reduce variation in plating. If one is not available, a multichannel pipette can be used. Just be sure to mix cells frequently as they can settle quickly.

4. Incubate cells at room temperature for 1 h.

   This helps to reduce a major source of variation in cell-based screening referred to as "plate effects", in which growth rates vary across wells of the plate [18].

5. Incubate the ES cells for 24 h at 37 °C and 5% CO_2.

   Using racks that allow for airflow between plates to allow for uniform temperature and CO2 levels helps to further reduce plate effects.

5   Compound Library and Screening

The labor involved in qRT-PCR-based screening prohibits very high throughput screens of hundreds of thousands of compounds. Libraries in the range of 10,000–50,000 are more suitable to the approach. Each 384-well plate should include unique compounds along with at least 24 wells for DMSO controls, 8–12 wells for positive controls (compounds or isolated cDNA), and 1–2 wells for no template control. It is critical to maintain positive and negative controls on every plate for accurate $-\Delta\Delta C_T$ calculations as well as proper assay quality control.

The screen requires manual set up at each step. With two people working side-by-side using the protocol and equipment described below, approximately forty 384-well plates can be processed during a typical 8-h day, completing a screen of 200 assay plates (30,000 compounds) in one week (*See* Fig. 4 for a depiction of the work flow). However, it is best to plan fewer plates (5–10) for the first few days until a good system is established. The use of liquid handlers and reagent dispensers makes this process much more robust and high throughput, although multichannel pipettes can and have been successfully used for small libraries or follow-up studies. If using multichannel pipettes, adjust the number of plates processed in a day accordingly.

A critical consideration before beginning is establishing the bookkeeping required during the two transfer steps. It is important to barcode all plates and keep careful records of source plates for all final qPCR plates.

1. Add test compounds (100 nl) to ~ 10 µM final concentration by pin transfer; each compound should be tested in duplicate.

   ES cells are particularly sensitive to DMSO concentration and it must be kept well below 1%. If a pin transfer tool is not available, it may be necessary to dilute compounds accordingly in PBS or media before adding them with a multichannel pipette or liquid handler.

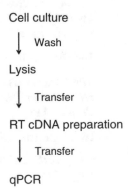

Fig. 4 A depiction of the workflow for the qRT-PCR high throughput screen. Note the two transfer steps that require careful record of source and destination plates

2. Incubate cells for 18 h at 37 °C and 5% CO_2.

3. Aspirate the media and wash cells with 100 μl PBS with a Biotek ELX405 plate washer.

   384-well plates can be difficult to aspirate without disrupting cells. It is important to verify in advance that any methods used to remove media are gentle enough to preserve cell integrity. It is also important to fully remove PBS after the washing step. We used a plate centrifuge to remove trace amounts of PBS by spinning plates upside down over paper towels at 50×g for 2 min.

4. Add 10 μl Cells-to-C_T™ lysis buffer containing DNaseI using a Thermo Multidrop™ Combi reagent dispenser. Agitate plates gently for 5 min at room temperature (19–25 °C) on a plate shaker.

   Do not overincubate as it can lead to RNA digestion.

5. Add Cells-to-C_T™stop solution (1 μl) using a Thermo Multidrop™ Combi reagent dispenser and incubate for 2 min at room temp (19–25 °C).

   Stop Point: *The lysis plates can be sealed and stored up to 6 months at −20 °C.*

6. Dispense 8 μl of Cells-to-C_T™ reverse transcriptase master mix into new PCR plates using a Thermo Multidrop™ Combi reagent dispenser

   The RT master mix is comprised of:

   5.0 μl 2× RT buffer.

   0.5 μl RT enzyme mix.

   2.5 μl nuclease-free water.

7. Transfer 2 μl of cell lysate into the PCR plate containing RT master mix using a CyBio® Well Vario and seal the plates with PCR film

8. Incubate the plates 37 °C for 60 min and then at 95 °C for 5 min in a PCR block.

   If screening many plates, this step can be a bottleneck. If that is the case, the 37 °C incubation can be performed in a standard incubator.

   Stop Point: *The cDNA can be frozen long term for years at -80 °C and used to detect other transcriptional targets.*

9. Dispense 4 μl qPCR master mix into 384-well qPCR plates.
   The qPCR master mix consists of:

   Roche Taqman® master mix (2.5 μl).

   40× FAM Bmi1 Taqman® probe (0.125 μl, Applied Biosystems).

   40× VIC actin Taqman® probe (0.125 μl, Applied Biosystems).

   Nuclease-free water (1.25 μl).

10. Add 1 µL cDNA from the RT reaction into the qPCR plate.

    At this point, if using isolated cDNA as a positive control, remove a row of tips from each box used for cDNA transfer corresponding to the wells designated for the positive control. At this point, also remove another two tips to provide a no template control to test for contamination.

11. Seal the plates with optical film.

12. Perform the qPCR run on the Roche Lightcycler 480 (or any 384-well compatible real time thermal cycler) with the following protocol.

    10 min incubation at 95 °C to activate the enzyme.

    40 cycles of 1 min at 60 °C and 15 s at 95 °C.

    The bottleneck for the screen is running the final qPCR plates. If only one machine is available, the maximum number of plates that can be run is 24 per day. However, the qPCR plates can be stored in the dark at 4°C for up to 2 weeks until all of the runs can be completed.

5.1 Data Analysis

1. Using the qPCR instrument software, generate a cycle call for when the sample enters log phase (C_T).

2. Calculate the fold change of *Bmi1* induction based on the $2^{-\Delta\Delta CT}$ calculations described by Livak and Schmittgen where $-\Delta\Delta C_T = (C_{T,\ Bmi1} - C_{T,\ Actin})_{Treated} - (C_{T,Bmi1} - C_{T,\ Actin})_{DMSO\ control}$ [17]. The "–delta delta C_T" values are calculated on a per plate basis using an average of the 24 neutral control (DMSO-treated) wells to account for plate-to-plate variation.

3. Establish a cutoff for hit calling. This cutoff is often determined after the screen is completed based on screen statistics (CV measurements and Z′ score) to ensure that hits are statistically significant and above the noise of the assay (usually at least three standard deviations above the mean). For example, we utilized a cutoff of 1.33 value for $-\Delta\Delta C_T$, which translated to a ~2.5-fold increase in *Bmi1* expression (50% induction of *Bmi1* levels compared to *Brg1* knockdown).

5.2 High-Throughput qRT-PCR Screen

We have observed excellent screening statistics using this protocol. CVs were comparable to those observed in the pilot screen, and excellent reproducibility was observed between replicates (Fig. 5). For our screen, a hit threshold of 2.5-fold increase or greater in *Bmi1* expression identified 98 compounds (final hit rate of 0.33%).

6 Confirmatory and Secondary Screens

6.1 Confirmation of Hits Using the Primary qRT-PCR Assay

Ideally the hits can be "cherry-picked" from dry powders and retested at a range of concentrations to determine dose responses. This smaller screen is run exactly as described above. We found

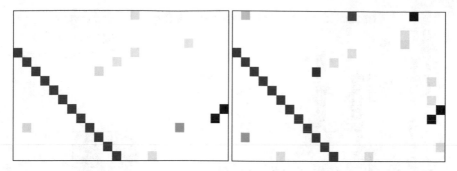

Fig. 5 An example of the high reproducibility between duplicate plates. Wells are depicted as a heatmap of the $-\Delta\Delta C_T$ values with darker colors corresponding to larger increases in *Bmi1* induction

that from 82 retested hits, 37 compounds produced a dose-dependent response in the qRT-PCR assay. The remaining compounds were eliminated due to lack of activity, lack of a dose-dependent response, or observed toxicity. This toxicity results in outliers with high actin C_T values and can often be eliminated after the primary screen.

6.2 Secondary Screen Using SYBR qRT-PCR

Next, confirm the ability of hit compounds to induce transcriptional changes using a SYBR-based qPCR assay system and a novel primer set. One of the benefits of a qRT-PCR screen is that the same cDNA can be utilized for all of the confimatory screens, as only 0.5–1 μl out of the 10 μl generated is required for each assay. For these screens we used the Roche SYBR master mix (2.5 μl 2× master mix, 1 μl cDNA, 0.5 μL primers (final concentration of 0.5 μM), and 1 μl nuclease-free water) and appropriate amplification conditions. We found that of 37 hits identified above, 34 induce *Bmi1* upregulation with the SYBR primer set.

6.3 Validation of Additional Transcriptional Targets

The ability to resample the cDNA samples obtained during the rescreen of hits for multiple relevant targets is a distinct advantage of the qRT-PCR approach. If screening for inhibitors of a transcriptional regulator, it is beneficial to identify how compounds affect the regulation of a panel of known target genes. In this manner, compounds that are acting on a separate target or pathway responsible for regulation of the target gene can be eliminated. If an option, it may be beneficial to test both activated and repressed target genes to eliminate compounds that may have general repressive activities. Following analysis of mRNA expression levels of seven additional BAF transcriptional targets (*Phox2b*, *Socs3*, *Eed*, *Ring1a*, *Cbx7*, *FGF4*, and *Bmp4*) 20 compounds out of 34 validated hits regulated these targets in a manner similar to BAF (Fig. 6) [6].

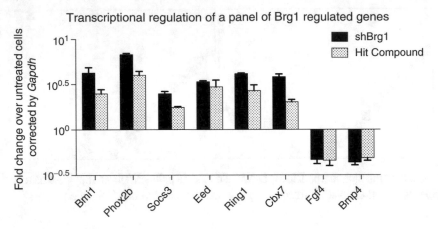

Fig. 6 A SYBR-based qRT-PCR secondary screen of additional targets of the transcriptional regulator BAF identifies 20 novel compounds that regulate gene expression in a manner similar to BAF deletion, as represented by knockdown of *Brg1*, the ATPase subunit

7 Conclusions

While qRT-PCR is still limited by price and throughput as an assay for high throughput screening, it provides distinct advantages in terms of robustness, reproducibility, and ease of setup. Here we provide a step-by-step protocol for optimizing and implementing a qRT-PCR screen in mouse embryonic stem cells that can be optimized in the time span of a few weeks. Using this system, it is relatively easy to screen libraries on the order of ten thousand compounds within a week and obtain highly reproducible data with few artifacts.

8 Resources

Bio-Rad: http://www.bio-rad.com/en-us/applications-technologies/qpcr-real-time-pcr

Ambion® Cells to C_T™ System: https://www.lifetechnologies.com/us/en/home/life-science/dna-rna-purification-analysis/rna-extraction/rna-types/total-rna-extraction/cells-to-ct-kits.html

Roche Lightcycler®: http://lifescience.roche.com/shop/en/ch/overviews/brand/real-time-pcr-overview

Life Technologies/Applied Biosystems Taqman® probes: http://www.lifetechnologies.com/us/en/home/life-science/pcr/real-time-pcr/real-time-pcr-assays.html

References

1. Eggert US (2013) The why and how of phenotypic small-molecule screens. Nat Chem Biol 9:206–209

2. Zhang Z, Guan N, Li T, Mais DE, Wang M (2012) Quality control of cell-based high-throughput drug screening. Acta Pharm Sin B 2:429–438

3. Auld DS, Thorne N, Nguyen D-T, Inglese J (2008) A specific mechanism for nonspecific activation in reporter-gene assays. ACS Chem Biol 3:463–470

4. Rao SSP et al (2014) A 3D map of the human genome at kilobase resolution reveals principles of chromatin looping. Cell 159:1665–1680

5. Kagey MH et al (2010) Mediator and cohesin connect gene expression and chromatin architecture. Nature 467:430–435

6. Ho L et al (2009) An embryonic stem cell chromatin remodeling complex, esBAF, is an essential component of the core pluripotency transcriptional network. Proc Natl Acad Sci 106:5187–5191

7. Dykhuizen EC, Carmody LC, Tolliday N, Crabtree GR, Palmer MAJ (2012) Screening for inhibitors of an essential chromatin remodeler in mouse embryonic stem cells by monitoring transcriptional regulation. J Biomol Screen 17:1221–1230

8. Ho L et al (2009) An embryonic stem cell chromatin remodeling complex, esBAF, is essential for embryonic stem cell self-renewal and pluripotency. Proc Natl Acad Sci 106:5181–5186

9. Wu J, Lessard J, Crabtree G (2009) Understanding the words of chromatin regulation. Cell 136:200–206

10. Kadoch C et al (2013) Proteomic and bioinformatic analysis of mammalian SWI/SNF complexes identifies extensive roles in human malignancy. Nat Genet 45:592–601

11. Bultman S, Gebuhr T, Magnuson T (2005) A Brg1 mutation that uncouples ATPase activity from chromatin remodeling reveals an essential role for SWI/SNF-related complexes in beta-globin expression and erythroid development. Gene Dev 19:2849–2861

12. Phelan M, Sif S, Narlikar G (1999) Reconstitution of a core chromatin remodeling complex from SWI/SNF subunits. Mol Cell 3(2):247–253

13. Ho L et al (2011) esBAF facilitates pluripotency by conditioning the genome for LIF/STAT3 signalling and by regulating polycomb function. Nat Cell Biol 13:903–913

14. Lessard J, Sauvageau G (2003) Bmi-1 determines the proliferative capacity of normal and leukaemic stem cells. Nature 423:255–260

15. Kreso A et al (2014) Self-renewal as a therapeutic target in human colorectal cancer. Nat Med 20:29–36

16. Bittker JA (2012) High-Throughput RT-PCR for small-molecule screening assays. Curr Protoc Chem Biol 4:49–63

17. Livak KJ, Schmittgen TD (2001) Analysis of relative gene expression data using real-time quantitative PCR and the $2-\Delta\Delta CT$ method. Methods 25(4):402–408

18. Lundholt BK, Scudder KM, Pagliaro L (2003) A simple technique for reducing edge effect in cell-based assays. J Biomol Screen 8(5):566–570

Chapter 7

Methods for MicroRNA Profiling in Cancer

Sushuma Yarlagadda, Anusha Thota, Ruchi Bansal, Jason Kwon, Murray Korc, and Janaiah Kota

Abstract

MicroRNAs (miRNA) are small non-coding RNAs that negatively regulate post-transcriptional gene expression. Almost all human cancers are characterized by abnormal microRNA expression patterns, which are unique to tumor types. A large body of experimental evidence documents the role of miRNAs in cancer pathogenesis, and specific miRNAs function as oncogenes or tumor suppressors. Due to unique expression profiles and anti/pro-tumorigenic properties of miRNAs, efforts are underway to explore their therapeutic and diagnostic potential. Many miRNA profiling methods have been developed, ranging from Northern blotting and qRT-PCR to the more recent microarray and RNA-Seq platforms. The following chapter details an imaging technique for cellular-specific miRNA expression profiling called in situ hybridization (ISH).

Key words MicroRNA, Expression profiling, Molecular imaging, ISH (in situ hybridization), Cancer

1 Introduction

MicroRNAs (miRNAs) are a group of conserved, small endogenous RNAs that function to post-transcriptionally regulate gene expression rather than encode protein. The gene inhibiting nature of miRNAs prompted their initial discovery in 1993 by Victor Ambros and his group during investigation of the *lin-4* gene, which is known to control larval development timing in *C. elegans* [1]. The team discovered that *lin-4* produces 18–25 nucleotide-long transcripts that directly or indirectly inhibit translation of *lin-14* messenger RNA (mRNA), thereby negatively regulating its protein expression levels. Seven years after the first miRNA discovery, Gary Ruvkun's laboratory identified a second miRNA, *let-7*, involved in *C. elegans* development [2]. Subsequently, three independent groups used a range of biochemical and cloning techniques and identified ~100 new miRNAs in *Drosophila, C. elegans,* and human genomes [3–5]. Since then, discovery of miRNAs has been rising exponentially. Over 6,400 mature human miRNAs are

Barbara Stefanska and David J. MacEwan (eds.), *Epigenetics and Gene Expression in Cancer, Inflammatory and Immune Diseases,* Methods in Pharmacology and Toxicology, DOI 10.1007/978-1-4939-6743-8_7, © Springer Science+Business Media LLC 2017 known to date, while projected numbers of all existing miRNAs reach much higher [6].

miRNAs are transcribed from individual genes containing their own promoters or intragenically from spliced portions of coding genes [7]. Similar to protein-coding genes, miRNA genes are transcribed by RNA polymerase II to produce a long primary transcript (pri-miRNA) that is 5′ methyl capped and has a 3′ polyadenylated tail [8]. A pri-miRNA transcript that can carry more than one mature miRNA is termed polycistronic miRNA transcript. The pri-miRNA is then processed inside the nucleus by RNase III endonuclease Drosha and cofactor DGCR8/Pasha to generate a 60–70 nt, stem-and-loop structure hairpin referred to as precursor miRNA (pre-miRNA) [9]. A double-stranded RNA-binding protein, known as exportin-5, then uses a RanGTP gradient to transport pre-miRNA from the nucleus to the cytoplasm for further processing and cleavage [10]. In the cytoplasm, pre-miRNAs are processed by another RNase III endonuclease, Dicer, to yield 20–23 nt double-stranded mature miRNAs [11]. One strand of the mature miRNA, called the passenger strand or miRNA*, is usually degraded and another called guide strand, that is incorporated into an Argonaut 2 protein complex called RNA-induced silencing complex (RISC) [12]. Refer to Fig. 1, illustrating an overview of miRNA biogenesis.

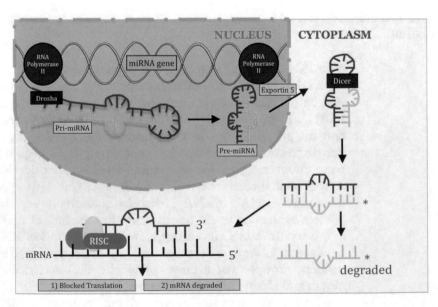

Fig. 1 miRNA biogenesis and function. pri-miRNAs are transcribed by RNA polymerase II and cleaved by Drosha to liberate the pre-miRNA that is transported to the cytoplasm by exportin 5. Dicer then performs a second cleavage event, generating a 21–23 nucleotide RNA duplex. One strand of this duplex is incorporated into the RNA-induced silencing complex (RISC) and guides silencing of target mRNA either by translational repression or degradation or both

Once the mature miRNAs are incorporated into the RISC complex, they guide the RISC complex to target mRNAs via antisense RNA-RNA interactions and regulate mRNA stability and/or translation. If the miRNA is highly complementary to its target transcript, degradation follows; when there is imperfect complementarity, translation is repressed or both [8, 13]. In either case, efficient recognition of target transcripts involves continuous base pairing between the first two to eight nucleotides in the 5′ end of miRNA (the seed sequence) and the 3′ UTR of its target mRNA [14]. miRNAs with identical seed sequences are considered family members [13, 15]. A single miRNA is capable of targeting hundreds of various transcripts associated with inter and intra cellular pathways [16]. Furthermore, a single mRNA transcript may be regulated by multiple miRNAs, whether they belong to the same family or are unrelated miRNAs with diverse target sites within a single transcript [17]. Thus, predictions indicate that miRNAs may regulate up to 30 % of encoding genes in humans [18].

This complex relationship between miRNAs and targets is critical in gene regulation and maintenance of cellular homeostasis. miRNAs are known to play a vital role in diverse cellular processes including development, metabolism, immune function, and response to external stimuli [19, 20]. As a consequence, disruption of miRNAs can have a profound impact on normal cellular physiology and could lead to disease. Accordingly, dysregulation of miRNAs has been well documented in almost every single human disease including cardiovascular defects, diabetes, and cancers [21, 22]. Among all the human diseases, the role of miRNAs in cancer pathogenesis has been cited extensively. In fact, more than half of the studied miRNA genes were found in cancer-associated genomic regions or fragile sites [23, 24]. miRNAs that regulate cell proliferation, differentiation, cell growth, survival, and apoptosis were found to have abnormal expression levels in various human cancers [25]. For example, loss of miR-15/16 limits the ability of the cell to inhibit anti-apoptotic gene *BCL2*, thereby promoting tumor progression; conversely, upregulation of miR-21 represses pro-apoptotic gene *PTEN*, promoting cell proliferation [26, 27]. Additionally, miRNAs are known to provide critical functions downstream of classic oncogenes and tumor suppressor signaling pathways such as Myc and p53 [28–31]. Consequently, potential therapeutic approaches that target miRNA pathways have recently attracted attention [32]. Some of the miRNA-based anti-cancer drugs are undergoing human clinical trials [33] or are in advanced phases of clinical product development [34–36].

In addition to their potential use as anti-cancer agents, abundant evidence supports the use of miRNAs as biomarkers for cancer diagnosis, prognosis, and treatment [37]. miRNAs remain intact and stable in various body fluids as well as in fixed and processed tissues, rendering them as ideal biomarkers for detection and quantification [38, 39]. Furthermore, studies suggest that serum/plasma levels of specific miRNAs correlate with the presence of hematologic malignancies and solid tumors, and are considered valuable markers for early detection of various cancer types [40].

Due to the important role of miRNAs in human malignancies and their potential use as anti-cancer agents and biomarkers, a number of miRNA identification and expression profiling/detection methods have been developed, each with their own advantages and disadvantages as listed in Table 1. For example, the role of miR-15/16 in chronic lymphocytic leukemia was discovered via positional cloning and forward genetics [41], similar to founder miRNAs *lin-4* [1] and *let-7* [2]. However, the vast majority of new miRNAs were discovered using small RNA libraries or RNA sequencing approaches [3]. To analyze expression of known miRNAs in tissues and body fluids, a wide variety of miRNA profiling methods such as Northern blotting, microarray, qRT-PCR, and in situ hybridization are routinely used. Identification and detection methods are generally chosen depending on the amount of tissue available for RNA isolation and the type of tissue or body fluid.

Northern blotting involves separation of small RNAs by size using polyacrylamide gels and hybridizing the blots with probes specific to miRNAs. In northern blot analysis, a known synthetic oligo ribonucleotide series is run alongside the samples for size determination. In addition, blots are probed with ubiquitously expressed small RNAs (U6, SnoRNA-Nucleus; tRNA-cytoplasm) to quantify the miRNA expression levels [42]. All microarray-based profiling methods utilize the simple Watson-Crick base pairing rules of nucleic acids. Known miRNA antisense probes are spotted onto a nylon support platform using machines/robotics. Test sample RNAs are hybridized with miRNA arrays and the expression levels are determined based on the specific miRNA probe signal intensity [43, 44]. Both Northern blots and microarrays are inexpensive. However, one major limitation is the need for large amounts of sample, an issue not pertinent to quantitative Reverse Transcription-Polymerase Chain Reaction (qRT-PCR).

In qRT-PCR, total RNA isolation is followed by polyadenylation and fractionation to enrich for miRNA transcripts. In addition, commercial kits are available to isolate small RNA fractions from total RNA. Unlike qRT-PCR for mRNA transcripts which involves poly (A) tails that are primed with poly (T)s and reverse transcribed to complimentary DNA (cDNAs), miRNA cDNA reactions are typically conducted using cDNA primers specific for each individual miRNA. Subsequently, the cDNA is amplified using miRNA-specific primers to quantify the miRNA expression levels. qRT-PCR is one of the few profiling methods capable of distinguishing between the precursor and mature miRNAs. The three primer miRNA probe/assay methods described previously are robust to

Table 1
An overview of miRNA expression profiling methods used in cancer research, with the advantages and disadvantages of each.

Method	Advantages	Disadvantages
Northern blotting	• Simple, reliable, and inexpensive • Provides size of the detected molecules • Efficiently validates newer profiling methods • Blots can be stored long-term and reprobed	• Laborious and sample-intensive • Requires high doses of radioactivity and formaldehyde • Risk of degradation during electrophoresis
Microarray	• Economical and commercially available • Various laboratories with different microarray platforms can compare and share data • Direct labeling of small RNA can be performed chemically or enzymatically • Can screen large numbers of miRNAs simultaneously	• Relatively lower specificity (compared to qRT-PCR and sequencing) • Using handheld spotting devices results in large arrays • Some require large RNA samples, reducing capability of sufficient sensitivity in profiling expression in small number of cells
qRT-PCR	• Can analyze small tissue samples • Used to validate predicted miRNAs • Highly sensitive and specific • Require low amounts of sample RNA • Differentiates between precursor & mature miRNAs	• Known miRNAs • Low-throughput
in situ	• Can visualize location of miRNAs within cells and between different cell types • Detects colocalization of at least 2 miRNAs and protein markers	• Proper fixation of small RNAs can be difficult • Time-consuming • Labor-intensive • Optimization made difficult by complicated workflow
Bead-based	• Economical and user-friendly • Superior statistical performance • Fast hybridization kinetics • High flexibility in array preparation • High specificity	• Labor-intensive • Requires PCR, hybridization, and optimized flow cytometer
RNA sequencing	• High sensitivity and accuracy • Size selection ensures enrichment for small RNAs • Can be used for discovery of unknown miRNAs	• Very expensive • Requires a lot of computational work during analysis of data
Cloning	• Reflect relative concentrations in a sample well • Powerful approach for unknown miRNAs • Can identify sequence variations, mutations, and single nucleotide polymorphisms associated with mature miRNA sequences	• Laborious • Systematic bias due to secondary structure of the different small RNAs that affect adapter ligation efficiency
Nano-technology	• Highly sensitive and specific	• Must be validated with another method to confirm expression levels

quantify the miRNA expression in RNA samples isolated from cells, body fluid, and tissues. However, miRNAs are expressed in a tissue- and cell-type-specific manner [45–47], and tumors are heterogeneous in nature [48–50]. To profile the miRNA expression in various cell types, an imaging-based method called in situ hybridization (ISH) is commonly employed in cancer research. Detailed below is the protocol for quantifying miRNA expression in formalin-fixed paraffin embedded (FFPE) tumor specimens via ISH [51]. This technique utilizes tyramide signal amplification (TSA) method allowing for the co-detection of more than one microRNA target via ISH and/or a protein marker via immunofluorescence [52].

2   Materials for In Situ Hybridization

NOTICE: Please *see* **Notes 1–9** in Subheading 4 prior to starting in situ hybridization.

1. **Fluorochrome Conjugated Tyramine Substrate**:
   (a) Fluorochrome-NHS ester solution: Fluorochrome-NHS ester is diluted at 10 mg/mL in dimethylformamide (DMF).
   (b) TEA solution: 1 % triethylamine (v/v) is diluted in DMF.
   (c) Tyramine solution: Tyramine hydrochloride is diluted at 10 mg/mL in TEA solution.
   (d) Tyramine solution is added to fluorochrome-NHS ester solution to make a solution of 1:1 molar ratio and is incubated on a shaker in the dark for 2 h.
   (e) The resulting 1:1 solution is diluted in equal volume of 100 % ethanol and stored at −20 °C. The resulting fluorochrome conjugated tyramine solution can be stored for at least 6 months.

2. **Diethyl Pyrocarbonate (DEPC)-Treated Water:** 1 mL of DEPC is added for every 1 L of double distilled water to make 0.1 % (v/v) DEPC-treated water (RNase-free water) and shaken vigorously. Resulting solution is incubated at 37 °C for 12 h and then autoclaved to 100 °C for 15 min.

3. **DEPC-Treated Glassware:** After washing with detergent, glassware is filled with 0.1 % DEPC in water and allowed to stand for 12 h at 37 °C. Then, glassware is autoclaved or heated to 100 °C for 15 min. The DEPC-treated water is decanted and glassware is dried in RNase-free area or a heated oven.

4. **20× Sodium Chloride-Sodium Citrate (SSC) Buffer Stock Solution:** 20× SSC powder is added to 1 L RNase-free water and shaken until dissolved.

5. **2× SSC Solution:** 25 mL of 20× SSC stock solution is added to 225 mL RNase-free water and stored at 4 °C.

6. **0.5× SSC Washing Solution:** 25 mL of 20× SSC stock solution is added to 975 mL RNase-free water and warmed to 55 °C (hybridization temperature).

7. **Ethanol Solution Series:** 247.5 mL of 200 proof ethanol is added to 2.5 mL RNase-free water for 99 % ethanol (v/v); 240 mL of ethanol is added to 10 mL RNase-free water for 96 % ethanol; 225 mL of ethanol is added to 25 mL RNase-free water for 90 % ethanol; 175 mL of ethanol is added to 75 mL RNase-free water for 70 % ethanol; 125 mL of ethanol is added to 125 mL RNase-free water for 50 % ethanol; 62.5 mL of ethanol is added to 187.5 mL RNase-free water for 25 % ethanol.

8. **Proteinase K Digestion Solution (5 µg/mL proteinase K in 10 mM Tris-Cl pH 8, 500 mM EDTA pH 8, and 50 mM NaCl):** 2.5 mL EDTA pH 8.0 and 2.5 mL 5 M NaCl is added to 2.5 mL of 1 M Tris-Cl pH 8.0 and mixed. The resulting solution is diluted in 242.5 mL RNase-free water (pre-warmed to 37 °C) and mixed. Finally, 62 µL proteinase K enzyme (20 mg/mL) is mixed into the solution and placed in a 37 °C incubator.

9. **1× Phosphate Buffered Saline (PBS) Solution:** 50 mL 20× PBS is added to 950 mL RNase-free water.

10. **0.2 % (w/v) Glycine Solution:** 400 mg glycine is added to 250 mL of 1× PBS.

11. **4 % (v/v) Paraformaldehyde (PFA) Solution:** 10 mL 20 % PFA is added to 40 mL of 1× PBS. 4 % PFA solution can be stored at 4 °C and used within a week.

12. **Acetylation Solution (66 mM HCl, 0.66 % acetic anhydride (v/v), and 1.5 % triethanolamine (v/v) in RNase-free water):** 16.6 mL HCl, 1.6 mL acetic anhydride, and 3.72 mL triethanolamine are added to 228 mL RNase-free water and shaken thoroughly. The solution is prepared in the chemical hood.

13. **Pre-hybridization Solution (50 % deionized formamide, 5× SSC, 1× Denhardt's solution, 500 µg/mL yeast tRNA):** 2.5 mL 20× SSC, 2 mL RNase-free DEPC-treated water, 500 µL RNase-free water containing 5 mg yeast tRNA, and 200 µL 50× Denhardt's solution are added to 5 mL formamide pre-warmed to 55 °C (hybridization temperature). The solution is prepared just before use and is placed at hybridization temperature.

14. **Hybridization Solution:** 9.6 μL LNA (250pmol) is added to 4.8 mL pre-hybridization solution and placed at hybridization temperature.

15. **Triton X-100 Solution (0.5 % Triton X-100 (v/v) in PBS):** 1.25 mL Triton X-100 is added to 250 mL 1× PBS and shaken.

16. **PBST Solution (0.02 % Tween*20 (v/v) in PBS):** 200 μL Tween*20 is added to 1000 mL 1× PBS and mixed thoroughly.

17. **H2O2 Solution (3 % H2O2 (v/v) in PBST):** 1 mL 30 % H_2O_2 is added to 9 mL 1× PBS.

18. **Blocking Solution (5 % bovine serum albumin (w/v) in PBST):** 500 mg Bovine Serum Albumin (BSA) is added to 10 mL PBST and shaken.

19. **PBT Solution (1 % BSA (w/v) and 0.1 % Tween*20 (v/v) in PBS):** 500 mg BSA and 50 μL Tween*20 are added to 50 mL 1× PBS and mixed well.

20. **TSA Solution (0.005 % H2O2 (v/v) in PBST):** 1 μL 30 % H_2O_2 is added to 20 mL PBST. The solution is prepared fresh.

21. **TSA Green Reaction Solution (1:200 stock fluorescein-conjugated tyramine in TSA solution):** 25 μL stock Fluorescein-Tyramine is added to 5 mL TSA solution. The solution is prepared fresh.

22. **TSA Blue Reaction Solution (1:500 stock AMCA-conjugated tyramine in TSA solution):** 10 μL stock Fluorescein-Tyramine is added to 5 mL TSA solution. The solution is prepared fresh (*see* **Note 10**).

23. **TSA Red Reaction Solution (1:1000 stock Rhodamine red-conjugated tyramine in TSA solution):** 5 μL stock Fluorescein-Tyramine is added to 5 mL TSA Solution. The solution is prepared fresh.

24. **MicroRNA Probes:** LNA probes were purchased from Exiqon. miR-29a LNA probe (3846715, Exiqon) is a 5′-digoxigenin (DIG) and 3′-DIG labeled probe whereas U6 snRNA LNA probe (9900203, Exiqon) is labeled with biotin at 5′ end.

25. **Antibodies:**

    (a) Mouse anti-DIG antibody conjugated to HRP solution (1:200 dilution of stock mouse anti-DIG (ab6212, Abcam) in PBT): 25 μL antibody is diluted in 5 mL PBT.

    (b) Streptavidin conjugated to HRP solution (1:5000 dilution of stock streptavidin conjugated to HRP (21130, Thermo Scientific) in PBT): 1 μL of stock streptavidin solution is diluted in 5 mL PBT solution.

(c) Rabbit anti-Actin Alpha 2 smooth Muscle (α-SMA) 1°
antibody solution (1:500 dilution of stock α-SMA antibody solution (NB600-531, Novus Biologicals) in PBT):
10 μL of stock α-SMA antibody solution is diluted in 5
mL PBT.

(d) Goat anti-rabbit IgG-HRP 2° antibody solution (1:500
dilution of stock goat anti-rabbit IgG-HRP (Santa Cruz,
sc-2004) antibody in PBT): 10 μL of stock goat anti-rabbit antibody solution is diluted in 5 mL PBT.

26. **Nuclear Marker** (Hoechst NucRedTM Dead647 #R37113,
Life Technologies): 10 drops of Hoechst NucRedTM Dead647
is added in 5 mL 1× PBS.

3   Method for In Situ Hybridization

This protocol is optimized for co-detection of miR-29a, snRNA
U6 and α-SMA (pancreatic stellate cell marker) in human PDAC
specimens as shown in Fig. 2 [51]. All steps are to be performed at
room temperature unless specified.

3.1 Deparaffinization and Rehydration of Tissue

1. The slides are baked at 65 °C for 30 min.

2. The slides are then cooled at room temperature for 5 min.

3. The tissues are deparaffinized by placing the slides four times
in xylenes for 5 min each.

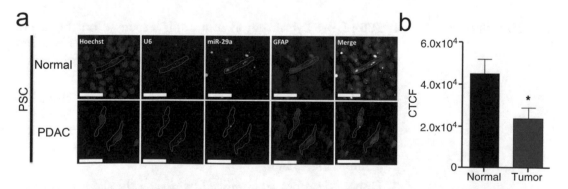

Fig. 2 miR-29 in-situ hybridization in SMA-positive pancreatic cells. (**a**) In situ hybridization of miR-29a in normal control and PDAC patient tumors. FFPE pancreatic tissue sections (5 μm) from normal control and PDAC patients ($n = 4$/group) were subjected to miR-29 *in situ* hybridization as described above in the protocol. Representative images are presented as a single channel, or merged (scale bar is 5 μm, 20× magnification). Hoechst Nuclear stain (*magenta*), positive control small nuclear RNA U6 (*red*), miR-29a (*green*), and PSC specific marker, Glial Fibrillary Acidic Protein (GFAP) (*blue*). (**b**) Corrected total cell fluorescence (CTCF) of miR-29a in PDAC tumors ($n = 4$) compared to control patients ($n = 4$) was calculated for GFAP-positive PSCs using ImageJ analysis as detailed in the protocol. Data represents mean ± S.E.M. Statistics were generated using *t*-test, *$p < 0.05$

4. The slides are transferred to 100 % ethanol followed by 99 % ethanol, 96 % ethanol, 90 % ethanol, 70 % ethanol, 50 % ethanol, and 25 % ethanol for 3 min each.

5. Slides are then rinsed in RNase-free water for 1 min.

6. Slides are washed three times in 1× PBS for 3 min each.

3.2 Proteinase K Digestion, Fixation, Acetylation, and Permeabilization of Tissues

1. Slides are placed in proteinase K digestion solution for 20 min at 37 °C (*see* **Note 11**).

2. The digestion is then stopped by incubating the slides in glycine solution for 1 min.

3. Slides are washed three times in 1× PBS for 3 min each.

4. The tissues are fixed with 4 % PFA solution for 10 min in the chemical hood (*see* **Note 12**).

5. After fixation, excess PFA is removed by washing the slides two times in 1× PBS for 3 min.

6. The slides are then transferred to acetylation solution in the chemical hood and incubated for 2 min.

7. The acetylation reaction is stopped by rinsing the slides in 1× PBS for 30 s followed by washing them two times in 1× PBS for 3 min each.

8. The cells are permeabilized by incubating them in Triton X-100 solution for 5 min.

9. Residual Triton X-100 is removed by rinsing the slides in PBS for 30 s followed by washing them three times in 1× PBS for 3 min each.

3.3 Hybridization

1. 200 µL pre-hybridization solution is dispensed on the top of the tissue sections and covered with parafilm strip. The slides are then incubated in a humidified chamber at hybridization temperature for 30 min (*see* **Notes 13** and **14**).

2. Residual pre-hybridization solution is shaken off (*see* **Note 15**) and 200 µL hybridization solution is dispensed on the top of the tissue sections and covered with parafilm strip. The slides are incubated in a humidified chamber at hybridization temperature for 90 min.

3. Unbound probes are removed by rinsing the slides in cold 2× SSC solution.

4. The slides are washed three times in 0.5× SSC solution for 10 min each at hybridization temperature.

5. The slides are either processed for TSA reactions after 15 min incubation in PBST solution or stored in PBST solution overnight at 4 °C.

3.4 TSA Green Reaction

1. The tissue sections are treated with 400 µL 3 % H_2O_2 solution for 15 min (*see* **Note 16**).

2. Then, the slides are washed three times in PBST for 3 min each.

3. 400 µL blocking solution is dispensed on the top of the tissues and incubated for 30 min.

4. Residual blocking solution is shaken off and the tissues are washed three times with 400 µL PBT for 3 min each.

5. Residual PBT is shaken off and 200 µL of anti-digoxigenin conjugated to HRP antibody solution is dispensed on the top of the tissue sections and covered with parafilm strip. The slides are incubated in a humidified chamber for 60 min.

6. Unbound antibodies are removed by washing the slides five times in PBST for 3 min each.

7. Residual PBST solution is shaken off and 200 µL TSA green reaction solution is dispensed on the top of the tissue sections. The slides are incubated in the humidified chamber for 20 min (*see* **Note 17**).

8. Excess TSA green reaction solution is removed by washing the slides five times in PBST for 3 min each.

9. The slides are either processed for the detection of the next marker after incubation in PBST for 15 min or stored in PBST solution overnight at 4 °C (*see* **Note 18**).

3.5 TSA Red Reaction

1. The tissue sections are treated with 400 µL 3 % H_2O_2 solution for 15 min (*see* **Note 16**).

2. Then, the slides are washed three times in PBST for 3 min each.

3. The tissues are washed two times with 400 µL PBT for 5 min each.

4. Residual PBT is shaken off from slides and 200 µL streptavidin conjugated to HRP solution is dispensed on the top of the tissue sections and covered with parafilm strip. The slides are incubated in a humidified chamber for 60 min.

5. Unbound streptavidin is removed by washing the slides five times in PBST for 3 min each.

6. Residual PBST solution is shaken off and 200 µL TSA red reaction solution is dispensed on the top of the tissue sections and incubated in a humidified chamber for 10 min.

7. Excess TSA red reaction solution is removed by washing the slides five times in PBST for 3 min each.

8. The slides are either processed for the detection of the next marker after incubation in PBST for 15 min or stored in PBST solution overnight at 4 °C (*see* **Note 18**).

3.6 TSA Blue Reaction

1. The tissue sections are treated with 400 μL 3 % H_2O_2 solution for 15 min (*see* **Note 16**).

2. Then, the slides are washed three times in PBST for 3 min each.

3. 400 μL blocking solution is dispensed on the top of the tissues and incubated for 30 min.

4. Residual blocking solution is shaken off and the tissues are washed three times with 400 μL PBT for 3 min each.

5. Residual PBT is shaken off and 200 μL of rabbit α-SMA 1° antibody solution is dispensed on the top of the tissue sections and covered with parafilm strip. The slides are incubated in a humidified chamber for 60 min.

6. Unbound 1° antibodies are removed by washing the slides five times in PBST for 3 min each.

7. Residual PBT is shaken off and 200 μL of goat anti-rabbit conjugated to HRP 2° antibody solution is dispensed on the top of the tissue sections and covered with parafilm strip. The slides are incubated in a humidified chamber for 45 min.

8. Residual PBST solution is shaken off and 200 μL TSA blue reaction solution is dispensed on the top of the tissue sections. The slides are incubated in the humidified chamber for 15 min.

9. Excess TSA blue reaction solution is removed by washing the slides five times in PBST for 3 min each.

10. The slides are either processed for the detection of the nuclear marker after incubation in PBST for 15 min or stored in PBST solution overnight at 4 °C (*see* **Note 18**).

3.7 Nuclear Marker Detection and Mounting of Slides

1. 200 μL of Hoechst NucRed™ Dead647 solution in 1× PBS is dispensed on the top of each slide and incubated in a humidified chamber for 10 min.

2. The slides are washed three times in 1× PBS for 15 min each.

3. The slides are then mounted with 20 μL ProLong Gold and sealed with glass cover slips.

4. Slides are usually allowed to cure overnight at 4 °C before proceeding to imaging and analysis under fluorescence microscope (*see* **Note 19**).

Microscopy and Image Acquisition: Images are acquired using CoolSNAP™ HQ2 CCD camera (Photometrics) mounted on a DeltaVision Core confocal microscope with fluorescent filter cubes AMCA/DAPI; fluorescein/FITC; rhodamine/TRITC; and hoechst647/CY5 using fluorescence insightSSI module (Applied Precision, #52-852113-003) equipped with 5 ms laser shuttering. Channels are acquired in grayscale; saved as .TIF files; and pseudocolored using SoftWoRx station. Respective channels are presented individually and merged as displayed in Fig. 2a. Although fluorescent insightSSI module was used for imaging in this protocol, any comparable fluorescence microscope with filters can acquire images of each fluorophore (fluorophore/excitation/emission: AMCA/381–412 nm/420–456 nm; FITC/464–492 nm/500–523 nm; rhodamine/531–565 nm/573–611 nm; hoechst647/619–646 nm/654–700 nm).

Quantification of Expression: The following is a modified version of a previously described protocol [53] and conducted using Image J software that is available for free (imagej.nih.gov/ij).

1. Utilizing α-SMA (or cell specific marker), outline the cell of interest using the free form selection tool, and copy/paste selection into new window.

2. Next, select *IMAGE* from the top toolbar, and select *Color*, then *Split Channel*.

3. Discard all other channels and keep the green channel image (or the channel corresponding to your miRNA of interest).

4. Select *ANALYZE* from the top toolbar, and select *Set Measurements* from the dropdown menu. From the pop-out menu check *AREA, INTEGRATED DENSITY,* and *MEAN GRAY VALUE.*

5. Again, select *ANALYZE* from the top toolbar and select *Measure* (or press ctrl + m). This will give a table of values (including *Area, Mean, Min, Max, IntDen* values).

6. Frequently, variability in background arises between slides. In order to subtract background and normalize signal measurements, select three or more regions adjacent/near your area of interest with no signal present. (NOTE: this will need to be repeated for every field of view).

7. Following the acquisition of measurements, copy and paste data into an excel sheet to calculate corrected total cell fluorescence (CTCF).

$$CTCF = Integrated\,Density - (\textit{Area of selected cell} \times \textit{Mean of background reading})$$

8. Repeat calculation for six or more cells and average CTCF values for each tissue section. Subsequently, graph the data in an appropriate graphical format that is desired.

4   Notes

1. All steps should be performed at room temperature unless mentioned.

2. Use RNase-free filtered tips for all steps.

3. Use DEPC-treated RNase-free double deionized water for all prehybridization and hybridization steps and SSC wash solutions.

Autoclaved Millipore water can be used for post-hybridization steps.

4. Treat pipetmen, glassware, working areas, and other objects to be used in the experiment with RNaseZap before conducting the experiment.

5. Read manufacturer's protocol and specification for each probe and antibody and alter protocol accordingly.

6. Adjust volumes of solutions according to the number of slides and as per requirement. The protocol above is designed for 24 slides.

7. Do not allow tissues to dry at any step as this will cause high background/false positive signal making it difficult to detect microRNAs and protein markers in dehydrated tissues.

8. Rinse the slides carefully but vigorously by dipping the slides 20 times before each incubation and washing step in coplin jars to equilibrate the solutions around the tissues.

9. The protocol is designed for FFPE tissues. It can be modified to be used in in vitro cells, but optimization is required. For in vitro cells, aspirate the media off the cells and wash twice in 1× PBS before conducting the experiment. Begin the protocol with fixation in 4 % PFA.

10. AMCA typically has a greater retention within tissues causing high background staining. In the event of high background staining, optimization of various dilutions of AMCA and added washes are recommended.

11. Some antibodies need an antigen retrieval step instead of proteinase K treatment to unmask the required antigen and restore the antigen-antibody binding. This needs to be optimized for each protein marker. For example, detection of CK19 using rabbit antihuman CK19 1° antibody (Abcam, ab52625) requires heat-induced antigen retrieval using citrate buffer at pH 6.0. This method does NOT require incubation in glycine following antigen retrieval.

12. Take care not to exceed 15 min in 4 % PFA during the fixation step, as prolonged fixation may cause masking of antigens.

13. This protocol is written for miR-29a *in situ* hybridization. User will need to optimize conditions for specific miRNA of interest. A temperature 20 °C below the Tm of miRNA(s) of interest is recommended as a starting temperature for hybridization temperature optimization in addition to ±5 °C. It is not recommended to go below 50 °C as this will result in precipitate formation in the prehybridization and hybridization solutions.

14. Use RNase-free water ONLY in humidified chambers during prehybridization and hybridization steps.

15. Following both prehybridization and hybridization steps, user is recommended to take precautions when removing the parafilm coverslips. Heated slides will tend to evaporate the applied solution more readily. Therefore, gently remove coverslips from each slide one at a time to avoid dehydration of slides.

16. Nonspecific signals can occur due to inadequate quenching of endogenous peroxidase enzyme. To resolve this problem, use a fresh bottle of 30 % H_2O_2 Stock Solution to prepare 3 % H_2O_2 and TSA Solutions.

17. Perform all post-hybridization steps starting with the first TSA reaction in the dark to avoid loss of signals from fluorochromes.

18. It is preferred if slides are incubated overnight before detection of the next marker so as to remove any excess residual TSA substrate to get a cleaner signal.

19. In the event of background signaling, increase SSC, PBST, and PBS washes to remove excess unbound probes, antibodies, or TSA substrates.

References

1. Lee RC, Feinbaum RL, Ambros V (1993) The C. elegans heterochronic gene lin-4 encodes small RNAs with antisense complementarity to lin-14. Cell 75(5):843–854

2. Reinhart BJ et al (2000) The 21-nucleotide let-7 RNA regulates developmental timing in Caenorhabditis elegans. Nature 403(6772): 901–906

3. Lagos-Quintana M et al (2001) Identification of novel genes coding for small expressed RNAs. Science 294(5543):853–858

4. Lau NC et al (2001) An abundant class of tiny RNAs with probable regulatory roles in Caenorhabditis elegans. Science 294(5543):858–862

5. Lee RC, Ambros V (2001) An extensive class of small RNAs in Caenorhabditis elegans. Science 294(5543):862–864

6. Londin E et al (2015) Analysis of 13 cell types reveals evidence for the expression of numerous novel primate- and tissue-specific microRNAs. Proc Natl Acad Sci U S A 112(10): E1106–E1115

7. Berezikov E (2011) Evolution of microRNA diversity and regulation in animals. Nat Rev Genet 12(12):846–860

8. Lee Y et al (2004) MicroRNA genes are transcribed by RNA polymerase II. EMBO J 23(20):4051–4060

9. Lee Y et al (2003) The nuclear RNase III Drosha initiates microRNA processing. Nature 425(6956):415–419

10. Yi R et al (2003) Exportin-5 mediates the nuclear export of pre-microRNAs and short hairpin RNAs. Genes Dev 17(24):3011–3016

11. Lee Y et al (2002) MicroRNA maturation: stepwise processing and subcellular localization. EMBO J 21(17):4663–4670

12. Hutvagner G, Zamore PD (2002) A microRNA in a multiple-turnover RNAi enzyme complex. Science 297(5589):2056–2060

13. Bartel DP (2009) MicroRNAs: target recognition and regulatory functions. Cell 136(2): 215–233

14. Wang X (2014) Composition of seed sequence is a major determinant of microRNA targeting patterns. Bioinformatics 30(10):1377–1383

15. Concepcion CP, Bonetti C, Ventura A (2012) The microRNA-17-92 family of microRNA clusters in development and disease. Cancer J 18(3):262–267

16. Lim LP et al (2005) Microarray analysis shows that some microRNAs downregulate large numbers of target mRNAs. Nature 433(7027):769–773

17. Krek A et al (2005) Combinatorial microRNA target predictions. Nat Genet 37(5):495–500

18. Lewis BP, Burge CB, Bartel DP (2005) Conserved seed pairing, often flanked by adenosines, indicates that thousands of human genes are microRNA targets. Cell 120(1):15–20

19. Bartel DP (2004) MicroRNAs: genomics, biogenesis, mechanism, and function. Cell 116(2):281–297

20. Rodriguez A et al (2007) Requirement of bic/microRNA-155 for normal immune function. Science 316(5824):608–611

21. Tijsen AJ, Pinto YM, Creemers EE (2012) Circulating microRNAs as diagnostic biomarkers for cardiovascular diseases. Am J Physiol Heart Circ Physiol 303(9):H1085–H1095

22. Karolina DS et al (2011) MicroRNA 144 impairs insulin signaling by inhibiting the expression of insulin receptor substrate 1 in type 2 diabetes mellitus. PLoS One 6(8), e22839

23. Munker R, Calin GA (2011) MicroRNA profiling in cancer. Clin Sci 121(4):141–158

24. Croce CM (2009) Causes and consequences of microRNA dysregulation in cancer. Nat Rev Genet 10(10):704–714

25. Calin GA, Croce CM (2006) MicroRNA signatures in human cancers. Nat Rev Cancer 6(11):857–866

26. Cimmino A et al (2005) miR-15 and miR-16 induce apoptosis by targeting BCL2. Proc Natl Acad Sci U S A 102(39):13944–13949

27. Zhang BG et al (2012) microRNA-21 promotes tumor proliferation and invasion in gastric cancer by targeting PTEN. Oncol Rep 27(4):1019–1026

28. O'Donnell KA et al (2005) c-Myc-regulated microRNAs modulate E2F1 expression. Nature 435(7043):839–843

29. Chang TC et al (2008) Widespread microRNA repression by Myc contributes to tumorigenesis. Nat Genet 40(1):43–50

30. He L et al (2007) microRNAs join the p53 network—another piece in the tumour-suppression puzzle. Nat Rev Cancer 7(11):819–822

31. Kota J et al (2009) Therapeutic microRNA delivery suppresses tumorigenesis in a murine liver cancer model. Cell 137(6):1005–1017

32. Orellana EA, Kasinski AL (2015) MicroRNAs in cancer: a historical perspective on the path from discovery to therapy. Cancers 7(3):1388–1405

33. Mirna T (2013) Mirna therapuetics is first to advance microRNA into the clinic for cancer. www.mirnarx.com. Accessed 13 May 2013

34. Daige CL et al (2014) Systemic delivery of a miR-34a mimic as a potential therapeutic for liver cancer. Mol Cancer Ther 13(10):2352–2360

35. Kasinski AL et al (2014) A combinatorial microRNA therapeutics approach to suppressing non-small cell lung cancer. Oncogene 34(27):3547–3555

36. Xue W et al (2014) Small RNA combination therapy for lung cancer. Proc Natl Acad Sci U S A 111(34):E3553–E3561

37. Iorio MV, Croce CM (2012) MicroRNA dysregulation in cancer: diagnostics, monitoring and therapeutics. A comprehensive review. EMBO Mol Med 4(3):143–159

38. Cortez MA et al (2011) MicroRNAs in body fluids—the mix of hormones and biomarkers. Nat Rev Clin Oncol 8(8):467–477

39. Boeri M et al (2011) MicroRNA signatures in tissues and plasma predict development and prognosis of computed tomography detected lung cancer. Proc Natl Acad Sci U S A 108(9):3713–3718

40. Allegra A et al (2012) Circulating microRNAs: new biomarkers in diagnosis, prognosis and treatment of cancer (review). Int J Oncol 41(6):1897–1912

41. Calin GA et al (2002) Frequent deletions and down-regulation of micro-RNA genes miR15 and miR16 at 13q14 in chronic lymphocytic leukemia. Proc Natl Acad Sci U S A 99(24):15524–15529

42. Iram S (2014) Northern hybridization: a proficient method for detection of small RNAs and microRNAs. Methods Mol Biol 1099:179–188

43. Babak T et al (2004) Probing microRNAs with microarrays: tissue specificity and functional inference. RNA 10(11):1813–1819

44. Nelson PT et al (2004) Microarray-based, high-throughput gene expression profiling of microRNAs. Nat Methods 1(2):155–161

45. Baskerville S, Bartel DP (2005) Microarray profiling of microRNAs reveals frequent coexpression with neighboring miRNAs and host genes. RNA 11(3):241–247

46. Landgraf P et al (2007) A mammalian microRNA expression atlas based on small RNA library sequencing. Cell 129(7):1401–1414

47. Hu G et al (2012) Identification of miRNA signatures during the differentiation of hESCs into retinal pigment epithelial cells. PLoS One 7(7), e37224

48. Meacham CE, Morrison SJ (2013) Tumour heterogeneity and cancer cell plasticity. Nature 501(7467):328–337

49. Marte B (2013) Tumour heterogeneity. Nature 501(7467):327

50. Junttila MR, de Sauvage FJ (2013) Influence of tumour micro-environment heterogeneity on therapeutic response. Nature 501(7467):346–354

51. Kwon JJ et al (2015) Pathophysiological role of microRNA-29 in pancreatic cancer stroma. Sci Rep 5:11450

52. Sempere LF et al (2010) Fluorescence-based codetection with protein markers reveals distinct cellular compartments for altered MicroRNA expression in solid tumors. Clin Cancer Res 16(16):4246–4255

53. Burgess A et al (2010) Loss of human Greatwall results in G2 arrest and multiple mitotic defects due to deregulation of the cyclin B-Cdc2/PP2A balance. Proc Natl Acad Sci U S A 107(28):12564–12569

Chapter 8

Microbiota and Epigenetic Regulation of Inflammatory Mediators

Marlene Remely, Heidrun Karlic, Irene Rebhan, Martina Greunz, and Alexander G. Haslberger

Abstract

Bacteria and bacterial derived metabolites are known to influence the host epigenetic regulation patterns such as DNA methylation and histone modifications, thus altering the expression of critical genes in pathologic processes, for example in metabolic syndrome. Fermentation end products, especially butyrate and LPS (lipopolysaccharides), the latter being cell-wall components of gram-negative bacteria, have been suggested as bioactive metabolites influencing epigenetic modifications by directly influencing enzymes catalyzing epigenetic modifications, by altering the availability of substrates, or by interactions with receptors. Thus, identification and quantification of gut microbiota via molecular based methods are of importance to address different epigenetic patterns and gene expression. We discuss methods for microbiota, epigenetic methylation, and expression analysis of our own research which will have a role in future studies.

Key words Microbiota and microbial epigenetic active products, Quantification of DNA and RNA, Gene expression analysis, Methylation analysis, Omics

Abbreviations

AMV	Avian myeloblastosis virus
APS	Ammonium persulfate solution
BGS	Bisulfite genomic sequencing
cDNA	Complementary DNA
DGGE	Denaturing gradient gel electrophoresis
DNMT1	DNA-methyltransferase 1
EDTA	Ethylenediaminetetraacetic acid
FRAR3	Free fatty acid receptor 3
FRET	Fluorescence resonance energy transfer
HDACs	Histone deacetylases
LPS	Lipopolysaccharide
5mC	5-methylcytosine
MeDIP	Methylated DNA immunoprecipitation

Barbara Stefanska and David J. MacEwan (eds.), *Epigenetics and Gene Expression in Cancer, Inflammatory and Immune Diseases*, Methods in Pharmacology and Toxicology, DOI 10.1007/978-1-4939-6743-8_8, © Springer Science+Business Media LLC 2017

MMLV   Moloney murine leukemia virus
MSRE   Methylation sensitive restriction enzyme
NF-kB   Nuclease factor kB
PTM   Posttranslational modification
qPCR   Quantitative real-time polymerase chain reaction
RT   Reverse transcription
SCFAs   Short chain fatty acids
SEM   Structural equation modelling
TE buffer Tris-EDTA buffer
TEMED N, N, N, N-tetramethylethylenediamine
TLR   Toll-like receptor

1   Analysis of Microbiota and Microbial Epigenetic Active Products

The gut microbiota has an important impact on digestion and metabolism of the host and plays an essential role in normal gut physiology [1]. Thus, a wide range of inflammatory and metabolic diseases are associated with microbial imbalance [2, 3]. Imbalanced gut microbial derived metabolites affect host epigenetic regulation patterns and consequently gene expression [4]. Butyrate and LPS (lipopolysaccharide) are the most common known microbial derived metabolites affecting DNA methylation and histone acetylation, which are key epigenetic markers in immune system modulation, energy extraction, and lipid metabolism. Potential mechanisms are the NF-kB (nuclease factor kB) signaling mediated from bacterial cell wall components [5] or the signaling via SCFAs (short chain fatty acids) produced by the microbiota. Many epigenetic modifying enzymes require nutrients or their metabolites as substrates or cofactors, thus dietary composition, bioactive nutrients, and gut microbiota composition are currently of research interest. An impaired ratio of *Firmicutes/Bacteroidetes* as well as SCFA-producers are shown to influence the promoter methylation of genes involved in inflammation (TLR2 (toll-like receptor), TLR4) [5] and fat metabolism (FFAR3 (free fatty acid receptor 3)) [6]. Thus, analysis of the gut microbiota diversity and composition of gut microbiota subpopulations, and the associated epigenetic patterns of gene expression are of high interest. For analysis of gut microbiota usually qPCR (quantitative real-time polymerase chain reaction) are used for compositional evaluation, for diversity analysis DGGE (denaturing gradient gel electrophoresis) is still the method of choice although microbial whole-genome sequencing facilitates mapping and comparing of genomes across multiple samples to generate reference genomes, microbial identification, or comparative genomic studies. Epigenetic patterns, such as DNA methylation within CpG dinucleotides, are verified after bisulfite conversion and pyrosequencing. Increase in DNA methylation within promoters and other regulatory gene regions is linked to gene silencing whereas decreased methylation within those regions correlates with overexpression [7].

1.1 Sample Preparation: DNA and RNA Extraction

High quality sample preparation is the first and most important step for every biomolecular analysis. Before starting the work, it is important to have standardized methods to obtain reproducible results. Implement the standards for a good laboratory practice, work carefully and methodically and, if necessary, repeat samples which do not maintain your requirements.

Nowadays there are a lot of companies who provide ready-to-use DNA and RNA purification kits. These kits enable genomic DNA and total RNA extraction from different sample types of humans, animals, plants, and bacteria. Some kits are nonspecific and some are specific for blood, tissue, stool, or cell samples and for only genomic DNA or RNA purification or simultaneous DNA/RNA purification. Depending on the needs, the type and origin of the sample, one should carefully choose a kit which meets requirements most.

The usage of commercial purification kits has some advantages. The standardized kits provide an optimized protocol, adjusted for different starting material to ensure high yields of DNA and RNA. The automated method can be beneficial in large studies to sustain reproducible results and extraction outcomes can be compared to other study results. Time can be saved on method development and optimization. However, disadvantages that have to be considered include chemicals and buffers of the kit, where the exact composition is not provided by the company, and specificity of the protocol can vary from supplier to supplier. Recently Dhaliwal (2013) published a list comparing commercially available extraction kits for different starting material [8].

Basically, main criteria for every DNA and RNA isolation method from any sample should include (1) efficient extraction, (2) sufficient amount of nucleic acids for further applications, (3) removal of contaminants, and (4) high quality and purity of DNA and RNA [8]. Figure 1 shows basic steps for every extraction method.

Commonly DNA and RNA have been extracted separately. Biomolecular analyses were simplified by simultaneous DNA and RNA extraction kits. Isolation of genomic DNA and total RNA from the same specimen has the advantage of providing matched nucleic acid fractions from the same cells, which is very beneficial for validations or integrative studies [9]. Therefore, when the amount of the sample is limited or when different analytical methods are carried out (e.g., endpoint PCR and real-time PCR) it is useful to extract both genomic DNA and RNA from the same sample. Then optimal comparison of for example gene expression and DNA methylation from a single biological sample is possible. Figure 2 shows steps for simultaneous DNA and RNA extraction methods.

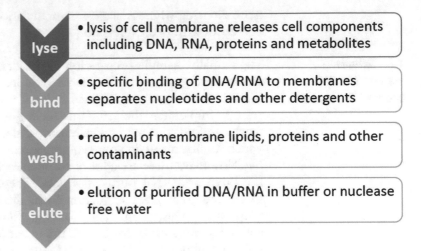

Fig. 1 Basic steps for every extraction method

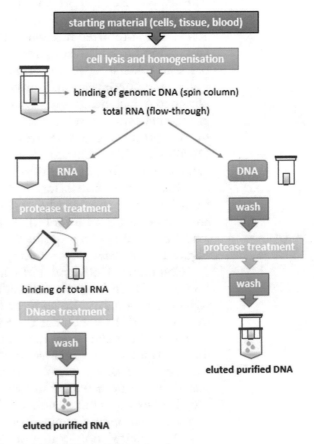

Fig. 2 Simultaneous DNA and RNA extraction

1.2 Purity Control of DNA and RNA

The concentration of DNA and RNA is typically measured with an UV/Vis Spectrophotometer. The absorbance of nucleic acid samples is quantified at 260 nm. At the same time, purity can be checked at ratios 260/280 and 260/230. The 260/280 ratio shows contamination with remaining proteins from extraction; for DNA a ratio ≥1.8 and for RNA≥2.0 should be achieved. Increased absorbance at 230 nm can show contamination as well. For pure samples the 260/230 ratio should be >2.0. A lower ratio can indicate contamination with different buffer salts. For example guanidine salts absorb between 220 and 230 nm. Guanidinium thiocyanate is commonly used in buffers for RNA purification. In this case, a ratio lower than 2.0 does not affect further processing.

As both RNA and DNA absorb at 260 nm and spectrophotometers do not discriminate between nucleic acids, RNA samples can be treated with DNase before measuring, to ensure there is no DNA contamination. UV/Vis tips, cuvettes and lenses have to be clean because this interferes with the absorbance and can alter the results. In addition, the measurement of the ratio 260/280 is pH-dependent [10]. Water can often be acidic and lower the 260/280 ratio. To assure correct readings a buffered solution with an alkaline pH, such as TE buffer (Tris-EDTA buffer, pH = 8.0), is recommended as diluent. The diluent has to be measured as blank for background corrections (http://www.lifetechnologies.com/at/en/home/references/ambion-tech-support/rna-isolation/tech-notes/quantitating-rna.html).

Agarose gel electrophoresis would be another method to check the purity and the product length after DNA/RNA extraction. Samples should have visible sharp bands (no smear bands) and the negative controls should be clean. The gels usually between 0.7 and 2 % dissolved in a suitable electrophoresis buffer are commonly stained and viewed under UV light.

1.3 Real-Time Polymerase Chain Reaction (qPCR)

Polymerase chain reaction is used, to amplify specific cDNA (complementary DNA) fragments with specific primers.

DNA denaturation: DNA is denatured at 95 °C into single strand. This temperature is held for a longer period of time to make sure DNA is separated properly and primers are not bound to DNA yet.

Primer annealing: Specific primers are annealed to single strand DNA at a primer-specific temperature. If temperature is to low, unspecific products can be the result, and if the temperature is too high, primers cannot anneal to DNA and no products can be formed.

Elongation: The enzyme *TaqPolymerase* binds to the 3′terminal end of the primers and completes the DNA strand complementary to the target sequence.

Table 1
PCR approach

Reagents	SYBR Green	TaqMan
Master mix	5 μL/sample	5 μL/sample
Primer (forward + reverse)	1 μL/sample	0.5 μL/sample
Probe	–	0.5 μL/sample
Nuclease-free water	1 μL/sample	1 μL/sample
DNA template	3 μL	3 μL
Total volume	10 μL	10 μL

There are different methods to measure DNA copies during PCR. Intercalating dye (e.g., SYBR Green or ethidium bromide), probes (e.g., TaqMan probe), or LUX (light upon extension) primers can be used. SYBR Green is an asymmetrical cyanine dye which binds to double stranded DNA. DNA–dye complex absorbs blue light (λmax = 497 nm) and emits green light (λmax = 520 nm). TaqMan technique uses 5′-3′ exonuclease activity of Taq-polymerase to cleave a so-called TaqMan-probe. A TaqMan-probe is an oligonucleotide which has two fluorophores, a reporter on the 5′-end and a quencher on the 3′-end. The quencher molecule quenches the fluorescence emitted by the reporter when energized by the cycler's light source via FRET (Fluorescence Resonance Energy Transfer). As long as these two fluorophores are together, there is no signal. Cleaving the reporter leads to a fluorescent signal which is measured in each cycle (Table 1).

Quantification can be made absolute or relative. In every cycle DNA is duplicated and measured. For absolute quantification standards with known concentrations are needed to calculate the amount of the gene sample. For relative quantification the target gene is compared to other genes, usually housekeeping genes (e.g., GAPDH, β-actin) with constant expression.

To check purity of reagents, all qPCR experiments should include a negative control (no-template, nuclease-free water). Further, in all SYBR-Green experiments a melt curve analysis is suggested to check correct annealing temperature and product quality.

1.4 Denaturing Gradient Gel Electrophoresis (DGGE)

DGGE is a molecular fingerprinting method. According to GC-content and melting temperature, endpoint PCR products of ribosomal subunit coding genes are separated in an acrylamide gel containing denaturing agent through a varying chemical gradient in an electric field. Sequences with a high GC content and higher melting temperature are located at the bottom of the gel whereas

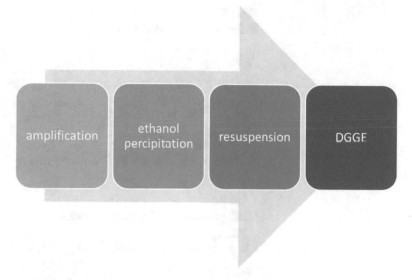

Fig. 3 Workflow for gut microbial diversity analysis

a low GC content in the sequence can be expected in the upper part of the denaturing gel. A separation is already possible with only one base difference, thus bacterial species can be separated and allocated on gel. The total bacterial diversity can be assumed with universal bacterial primers of 16S rRNA, which helps to estimate the richness of predominant gut microbiota [11]. Figure 3 shows the basic steps of diversity analysis with DGGE.

1.4.1 Amplification

After amplification of 16S rRNA with a ready-to-use GoTaq® Green Master Mix (Promega) with 1.5 mM MgCl$_2$ and the specific primer for total bacterial abundance 341f-GC 5'-CCT ACG GGA GGC AGC AG-3' [11] and 518r 5'-ATT ACC GCG GCT GCT GG-3' [12] (Table 2), assays are carried out in a 96-well Gradient Thermal Cycler (Labnet MultiGene™). A reference marker for total bacteria including fragments of 16S rRNA genes from cultured bacteria and clones generated from fecal material (e.g., *Bacteroides thetaiotaomicron*, *Enterococcus faecium*, *Clostridium leptum 16*, *Escherichia coli*, *Clostridium coccoides 43*, *Lactobacillus reuterii*, and *Bifidobacterium longum*) facilitates mapping.

1.4.2 Ethanol Precipitation and Resuspension

Precipitation takes place with 1 mL ethanol at −20 °C overnight. After 30 min. centrifugation at $14,000 \times g$ a pellet is shown at the bottom of the tube. To guarantee total liquid removal, a drying period at 30 °C shall be interposed before resuspension with loading part (5 μL) and nuclease-free water (15 μL).

1.4.3 DGGE Gel Preparation

According to Table 3 an 80 % and a 0 % solution has to be prepared to allow gradient preparation in gel. The gradient has to be selected according to estimated GC-content and melting temperature. For

Table 2
Endpoint PCR approach for DGGE

GoTaq® Green Master Mix (Promega)	50 μL/sample
Primer (forward + reverse)	1 μL/sample
BSA (bovines serum albumin)	2 μL/sample
Nuclease-free water	41 μL/sample
DNA	5 μL/sample

Table 3
DGGE gel solutions for gel preparation

80% Solution	0% Solution
40.5 g urea	
48 mL formamide	
30 mL acrylamide 40 %	40 mL acrylamide 30 %
1.5 mL TAE	1.5 mL TAE
Refill with H_2O up to 150 mL	Refill with H_2O up to 150 mL

total bacteria a linear gradient of 25–65 % is used. The chain reaction of polymerization from acrylamide to polyacrylamide is initiated by the radical APS (ammonium Persulfate Solution, 0.1 g in 1 mL nuclease-free water) and catalyzed by TEMED (N,N,N,N-tetramethylethylenediamine). The gel shall be refilled with the 0% solution at the comb position according to Muyzer et al. [13]. Polymerization needs about 1 day.

1.4.4 DGGE   DGGE gels shall be preheated to 60 °C before loading with Hamilton pipette. Volt, temperature, and time must be chosen accordingly, for total bacterial abundance: 175 V, 60 °C, and 6 h are used. After electrophoresis gels are stained and viewed under UV light.

2   Analysis of Gene Expression

The usage of a kit for DNA/RNA extraction will depend on the starting material and the priorities specified by the user. When working with whole blood, there are a few things to consider. To avoid coagulation, whole blood samples should be collected in the presence of an anticoagulant. For bioanalytical applications heparin coated tubes are widely used for blood collection, but heparin has been shown to interfere with DNA polymerase activity in PCR and real-time PCR [14, 15]. Therefore, EDTA (Ethylenediamintetraacetic acid) or citrate should be the anticoagulant of choice when following processes include real-time PCR. Anticoagulation tubes for blood collection are commercially available but can also be prepared in-house, especially when the expected or needed blood volume is less than the volume recommended for commercial tubes. To avoid coagulation of the blood a final ratio of 1.5–2.2 mg EDTA per 1 mL of blood should be used [16]. Therefore a stock solution of 18–20 mg K_2EDTA [17] or Na_2EDTA per 1 mL of distilled water can be prepared. Right before puncture, the syringe has to be treated with the EDTA solution by performing a couple of passages through syringe and needle to avoid clotting during blood collection. Immediately, add 10 % of the stock solution to the volume collected. After blood collection, samples should be processed within a few hours to ensure RNA stability. Immediate lysis and homogenization is effective to prevent RNA from degradation. Only homogenized blood samples can be stored at −70 °C for several months before RNA extraction. Depending on the kit, with only 200 μL of blood representative amounts of genomic DNA and RNA for following procedures can be achieved.

To protect tissue from RNA degradation, fresh samples should immediately be treated with RNAlater. Tissue can be stored in RNAlater at −80 °C for later extractions without loss of DNA or RNA yields.

2.1 Sample Processing: RNA

For gene expression analysis mRNA has to be converted into cDNA via the enzyme reverse transcriptase.

Biochemical enzymatic activities include RNA-dependent DNA polymerase activity which transcribes a RNA–DNA hybrid from an RNA template (reverse transcription; RT) and RNaseH activity which degrades the RNA from the RNA–DNA hybrid to produce single-stranded cDNA. cDNA is intron free, compared to genomic DNA (Fig. 4).

Commonly used RT enzymes are derived from different retroviruses such as avian myeloblastosis virus (AMV) and moloney murine leukemia virus (MMLV). These vary in different enzymatic activities. The RNA-dependent DNA polymerase needs primers to bind on RNA. These can be specific primers, random hexamers, or oligo-dT primers. Gene-specific primers decrease background priming, whereas the use of unspecific primers can maximize the cDNA molecules that can be analyzed [18], making it possible to get multiple information from one single sample. For complete

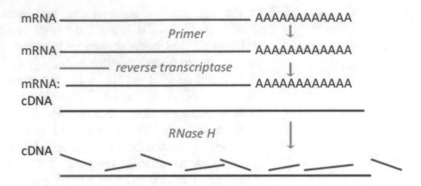

Fig. 4 Steps of reverse transcription

transcription the recommended amount of RNA should not be exceeded. Otherwise nontranscribed RNA can remain in the sample, which may affect following real-time PCR.

Quantification of cDNA is difficult with common UV–Vis Spectrophotometer. Left over products from RT interfere with the measurement leaving no reliable results. It is recommended to measure RNA after extraction and use a known amount for RT. Calculate the outcome and insert the needed concentration in real-time PCR. cDNA should be aliquoted to multiple tubes and stored at −80 °C. Refreezing and thawing affects the stability of cDNA.

3   Analysis of Epigenetic Modifications

The most important components of the epigenome which are commonly altered are (1) DNA-methylation, (2) histone modifications, and (3) microRNAs.

DNA methylation occurs mainly at cytosines within CpG (cytosine phosphorylated guanosine) dinucleotides in promoter regions and other regulatory regions. When a gene is being transcribed, RNA polymerase first has to bind to its promoter. However, it is sterically inhibited if cytosines at CpGs are methylated. In tumor cells, promoters of tumor suppressor genes are often hypermethylated, which leads to gene silencing. DNA methylation is catalyzed by DNA methyltransferases (DNMTs) including DNMT1 that is responsible for the maintenance of methylation patterns during replication.

Histone modifications include acetylation, methylation, phosphorylation, and ubiquitination, among others. The most studied one is acetylation and deacetylation which control the status of chromatin: which can be condensed (heterochromatin) or relaxed (euchromatin) and thus affect gene transcription. HDACs (histone deacetylases) are able to remove an acetyl-group from a histone tail, which results in a positively charged lysine. This lysine interacts

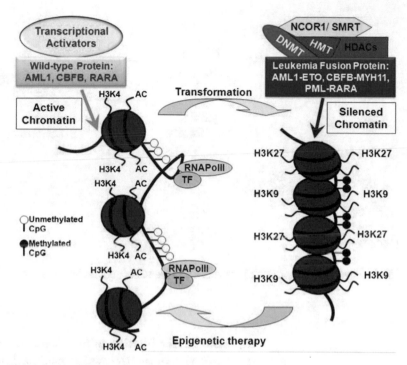

Fig. 5 Switching between euchromatin (*left*) and heterochromatin (*right*)

with a negative charged phosphate-group of a DNA strand which condenses chromatin (Fig. 5).

Micro RNAs were first described in 1993, but the name microRNA was first defined in 2001. As the name tells, these molecules are very short consisting of 20–25 nucleotides. MicroRNAs are a class of non-protein coding RNAs regulating gene expression posttranscriptionally in eukaryotes. After processing to a final effector form, they pair to the 3′ untranslated region (3′ UTR) of target mRNA, thus inhibiting transcription. Over 1000 miRNAs have been found in the human genome [19] rendering miRNAs one of the largest classes of regulatory molecules. Over a dozen miRNAs have been found to be induced by c-Myc to manifest its function in cell cycle, survival, metabolism, apoptosis, and metastasis [20]. To present an example, microRNA-137 promoter methylation in oral rinses from patients with squamous cell carcinoma of the head and neck is associated with gender and body mass index 25–30 kg/m_2 [21, 22].

3.1 Sample Processing: DNA

DNA methylation is a mechanism that alters gene expression. Methylation of CpGs in the promoter region of genes influences their transcriptional regulation. Hypermethylation and hypomethylation can silence or promote gene expression, respectively. Methylation at response elements is usually identified to constrain

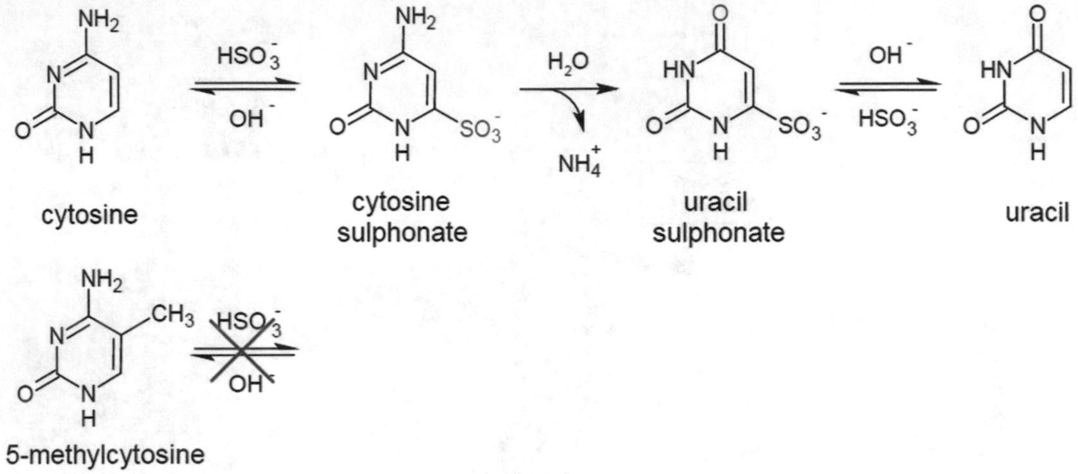

Fig. 6 Conversion of cytosine to uracil in the presence of sodium bisulfite

expression as the binding of promoters by transcription factors and other proteins of the transcriptional machinery is affected.

Methylation status of CpGs can be detected via sequencing, but first the DNA has to be bisulfite treated or a methylated DNA immunoprecipitation (MeDIP) is used as a purification technique to enrich methylated DNA sequences. Methylated DNA fragments are pulled by an antibody against 5-methylcytosine (5-mC). After sonication and denaturation DNA fragments (300–1000 bp) are bound by 5-mC antibody and conjugated to anti-mouse-IgG. Unbound DNA is removed in the supernatant. For DNA purification and release, proteinase K is added to digest the antibodies. DNA microarrays (MeDIP-chip) or next-generation sequencing (MeDIP-seq) are commonly used in combination with immunoprecipitation.

Due to bisulfite conversion unmethylated cytosines are fully converted into uracil in denatured DNA strands. High sodium bisulfite salt concentrations, high temperatures, and a low pH lead to the deamination of unmethylated cytosines into uracils. Figure 6 shows conversion from cytosine to uracil in the presence of sodium bisulfite.

3.2 Detection of Promoter-Specific Methylation Status: Pyrosequencing

In methylation analysis, usually CpGs in promoter regions are the target of interest because it is very likely that epigenetic changes in these regions lead to alterations in gene expression.

The database ensembl (http://www.ensembl.org/index.html) can be used to find the first exon and the promoter region of a gene. As an example, promoter region and first exon (red) of TNFα (mus muculus) with marked TATA-box and CpGs is presented:

GCTTTCAGAAGCACCCCCCCATGCTAAGTTCTCCCCCATGGATGTCCCATT

TAGAAATCAAAAGGAAATAGACACAGGCATGGTCTTTCTACAAAGAAAC

AGACAATGATTAGCTCTGGAGGACAGAGAAGAAATGGGTTTCAGTTCTCA

GGGTCCTATACAACACACACACACACACACACACACACACACACACACAC

ACACCCTCCTGATTGGCCCCAGATTGCCACAGAATCCTGGTGGGGACGAC

GGGGAGGAGATTCCTTGATGCCTGGGTGTCCCCAACTTTCCAAACCCTCTG

CCCCCGCGATGGAGAAGAAACCGAGACAGAGGTGTAGGGCCACTACCGC

TTCCTCCACATGAGATCATGGTTTTCTCCACCAAGGAAGTTTTCCGAGGGT

TGAATGAGAGCTTTTCCCCGCCCTCTTCCCCAAGGGCTATAAAGGCGGCC

GTCTGCACAGCCAGCCAGCAGAAGCTCCCTCAGCGAGGACAGCAAGGGA

CTAGCCAGGAGGGAGAACAGAAACTCCAGAACATCTTGGAAATAGCTCC

CAGAAAAGCAAGCAGCCAACCAGGCAGGTTCTGTCCCTTTCACTCACTGG

CCCAAGGCGCCACATCTCCCTCCAGAAAAGACACCATGAGCACAGAAAG

CATGATCCGCGACGTGGAACTGGCAGAAGAGGCACTCCCCCAAAAGATG

GGGGGCTTCCAGAACTCCAGGCGGTGCCTATGTCTCAGCCTCTTCTCATTC

CTGCTTGTGGCAGGGGCCACCACGCTCTTCTGTCTACTGAACTTCGGGGTG

ATCGGTCCCCAAAGGGATGAGGTGAGTGTCTGGGCAACCCTTATTCTCGC

TCACAAGCAAAACGGGTTAGGAGGGCAAGAAGGACAGTGTGAGGGAAAG

AAGTGGGCTAATGGGCAGGGCAAGGTGGAGGAGAGTGTGGAGGGGACAG

AGTCAGGACCTCGGACCCAT

For optimal sequencing conditions DNA samples have to be multiplied with end-point PCR. A forward primer, a reverse primer and a sequencing primer for subsequent sequencing are needed. Primers can be self-designed with programs available from commercial suppliers and ideally with matching programs for your sequencing method. The purity and the success of the PCR can be checked on agarose gel. Samples should have visible sharp bands (no smear bands) and the negative controls should be clean. Sometimes primer clouds can appear at the bottom of the gel. This means that primers were used in excess and need to be reduced.

The method of choice for gene specific methylation analysis is pyrosequencing. It is based on de novo DNA sequencing. If a nucleobase is attached by the polymerase, pyrophosphate is set free.

Through a cascade of enzymatic reactions a detectable light is generated. Single stranded, bisulfite converted DNA is amplified with a sequencing primer. An enzyme substrate mix is added to the reaction and the polymerase attaches to the strand. If an offered nucleotide is successfully built in, pyrophosphate (PPi) is set free. Through ATP-sulfurylase and PPi, dATP is generated from dADP. In the presence of dATP and luciferase, luciferin is oxidated to oxyluciferin and in this reaction light is released and can be measured at 560 nm. The intensity of the light is displayed in a so-called pyrogram.

In CpG analysis the sequence of interest is already known and sequencing is done in the known order, except for the CpG sites. If the cytosine was converted to thymine, it means the site was unmethylated. There are programs for CpG analysis where you detect either a C or a T in a CpG site and you can also control if the bisulfite treatment was successful by trying to detect a C (in non CpG sites) in front or after a T, which was a C before bisulfite treatment. Results of the analysis will be displayed in a pyrogram and CpG methylation status is shown in percentage (Fig. 7).

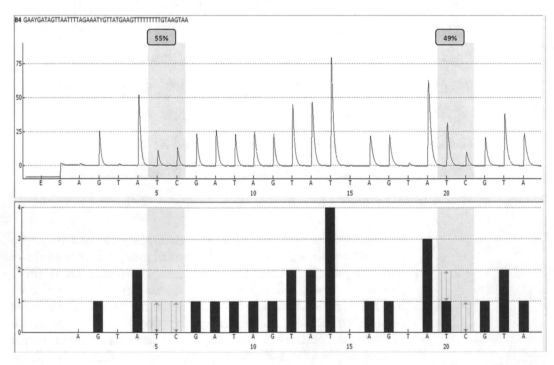

Fig. 7 Pyrogram of murine IL-6 CpG assay: The sequence to analyze is shown at the top (GAAYGATAGTTAATTTTAGAAATYGTTATGAAGTTTTTTTTTTGTAAGTAA). The histogram shows the dispensation order and the expected height of the peaks. Variable positions, to analyze methylation status of CpGs, are highlighted in blue background color. The methylation level of each CpG is shown as percentage in the Pyrogram (A, T, C, G = nucleotides, E = enzyme, S = substrate)

3.3 High-Throughput Analysis of Epigenetic Modifications

At prominent European Institution for validating biomarkers such as the Austrian Institute of Technology (AIT), top markers are derived from MEDIP-Seq in TwinsUK using "Bisulfite genomic sequencing" (BGS).

Evaluation is performed by bioinformatics of BGS data using the XworX workflow based software-framework for pipelined computing. For BGS confirmed markers, either bisulfite or methylation sensitive restriction enzyme (MSRE) based qPCRs-methodology are applied in a validation step. Compared to bisulfite based PCR approaches this MSRE-strategy enables validation of ten times more markers on the same amount of input DNA and is also very cost efficient. In addition, there is the possibility to validate markers using novel high throughput multiplex methylation analysis based on qPCR that is implemented and used for highly accurate, cost- efficient profiling. The technique is based on the competitive PCR approach developed at AIT [23–25] using the ultra-high qPCR platforms BIOMARK and OpenArray.

Genomic DNA is extracted from the blood or tissue samples collected from the subjects. The DNA is treated chemically with bisulfite to specifically convert non-methylated cytosines to uracil, while leaving methylated cytosines unchanged. The material is then aliquoted in the particular high throughput qPCR platforms and analyzed in a vast number of parallel competitive PCRs that each is designed such that the prevalent epigenetic form is preferably amplified and thus identified. By doing this it will be possible to confirm up to 96 predictive epigenetic biomarkers in up to 10,000 samples. The combination of the latest spotting techniques, fully robotized platform and new optical reading systems, AXO Science HIFI Technology, opened a new era in the large scale screening of several parameters for numerous patients (Fig. 8 and 9; more about AXO Science HIFI Technology at www.axoscience.com).

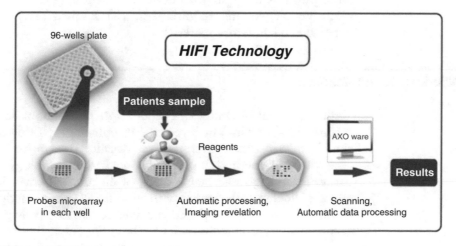

Fig. 8 AXO Science HIFI Technology overview

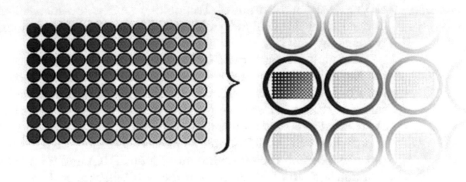

Classic 96 microwell plate   AXO Science plate

Fig. 9 AXO Science HIFI Technology plates

3.3.1 HIFI Technology Shows Several Assets

Fully robotized platform for multiplexed high-throughput assays can be adapted to any DNA, protein and peptide based assays. Up to 100 molecular probes can be immobilized in each well of classical 96 or 384 wells format. Other advantages include: processability in any automated laboratory system, cost effectiveness, optical detection of the positive results, quantitative detection of the level of interactions on each spot, protocol increasing the interactions between targets and immobilized probes and lowering the assay background. AXO Science HIFI Technology can be adapted to many molecular based diagnostic applications (blood genotyping, cancer diagnostic, pathogen detection, etc.).

Multiplexed assays bring the ability to profile multiple molecules from a single sample, in a single assay and are the next generation of bioanalytical systems. They offer many advantages: (1) Generate more information on interrelationships between related analytes within a sample with better correlation; (2) Decrease precious sample volume requirement; (3) Reduce assay reagent, expense and laboratory material.

4 Whole Genome Approaches

With the advent of Omics and other High Throughput Screening technologies, our insight into the pathophysiology of disease has significantly increased over the last decade. Integrative research concepts and methodologies such as Systems Biology geared towards deriving molecular models of disease. Systems Medicine aimed at linking such models with clinical and other descriptors of disease phenotypes. It opened the avenue towards truly grasping complexity of chronic diseases. On the other hand, these developments revealed major shortcomings in predicting clinically relevant outcomes such as diagnosis, prognosis, and rarely influence treatment decisions. Currently, complex molecular information at the individual patient level still has limited clinical utility.

An established platform for DNA methylome analysis is Illumina Infinium HumanMethylation450. This technology is an extension of the previous HumanMethylation27 BeadChip and allows us to assess more than 480,000 cytosines across the genome per sample. Twelve samples per chip and 4–8 chips (total of 48–96 samples) can be processed simultaneously. The platform incorporates two different probe types using different assay designs (InfiniumI and InfiniumII), which introduces technical variation and complicates the analysis process [26]. However, the application of this platform is continuously improving [27, 28].

4.1 Combination of Methylation and Histone Analyses

(For details see: http://blueprint.genomatix.de/).

This is currently investigated by the BLUEPRINT project, which was initiated in the fall of 2011, celebrated its first data release April 2012 when 12 full epigenomes of neutrophils and monocytes from both adult blood and cord blood became available through different data portals including the ENSEMBL and UCSC7 browsers, BIOMART8 and a visual interface developed by GENOMATIX. For each sample, the release included information on 6 IHEC recommended informative histone modifications (H3K4me1, H3K4me3, H3K27ac, H3K36me3, H3K9me3, and H3K27me3), DNA methylation at base pair resolution, RNA expression, and genome-wide accessibility through DNAseI-seq analysis. Future releases will also include epigenomic data on differentiation pathways, such as monocyte to macrophage and B-cell differentiation, and from more rare cell types from healthy donors as well as on diseased cell types. As an epigenomic project specifically focusing on hematopoiesis, BLUEPRINT is expected to make a major contribution to the field of blood epigenetics. The epigenomic maps generated within BLUEPRINT will provide comprehensive indexes of chromatin organization and associated functionality that will serve as an entry point for further investigations into the key transcription factors and regulatory networks that establish, regulate or maintain epigenomic features. Within one cell type, the epigenomic maps will allow the identification of gene classes with similar patterns of epigenetic features. That likely represents clusters with coordinated regulation of gene expression. Upon systematic comparisons between cell types, clusters of genes may prove to be coordinately regulated by epigenetic mechanisms throughout the hematopoietic differentiation program. In addition, chromatin state maps identification will allow assignment of the functional states (such as active, inactive, or poised) based on epigenetic profiles. The analysis will divide the genome into epigenetic segments comprising combinations of different epigenetic features such as DNA methylation, histone modifications and accessibility, and relate these to function. The identification of such segments and comparison with perturbed epigenetic landscapes in disease will trigger investigations into the restoration or repair of the epigenetic code of these elements [29, 30].

4.2 Pathway Analysis and Statistical Modelling

Pathway Analysis and statistical modelling is utilized to examine the genomic, metabolomic, and PTM (posttranslational modification) data in a biologically relevant manner. The molecules represented in our metabolomic, methylome, and genome data for birthweight that are also associated with aging phenotypes, will be annotated and converted to human identifiers using public-access tools and assigned to pathways with the GeneGo MetaCore program (www.genego.com). This program assigns pathway significance based upon the number of genes represented within a pathway and the direction of change. The overwhelming benefit to this methodology is that change in a single gene will be ignored unless related genes also demonstrate an altered pattern (genetic association/methylation/metabolite abundance). This type of analysis allows integration of the typical genomic/metabolomic methodology with the systems biology approaches of examining large numbers of genes, some of which may be expressed only at low levels despite their importance to a given pathway [31]. In addition, to identify mediators or modifiers of the top genetic variants, metabolomic, epigenetic and PTM associations over the life course, appropriate statistical methods for dealing with complex relations, such as structural equation modelling (SEM) and/or Bayesian approaches, will be applied. Current studies aim to obtain more information on the networks of variables that have an impact along the life course and gain a better understanding of the mechanisms by which genetics and epigenetics play a role in health associated phenotypes.

References

1. Aziz Q, Doré J, Emmanuel A, Guarner F, Quigley EM (2013) Gut microbiota and gastrointestinal health: current concepts and future directions. Neurogastroenterol Motil 25(1):4–15
2. Larsen N, Vogensen FK, van den Berg FW, Nielsen DS, Andreasen AS, Pedersen BK, Al-Soud WA, Sorensen SJ, Hansen LH, Jakobsen M (2010) Gut microbiota in human adults with type 2 diabetes differs from non-diabetic adults. PLoS One 5(2), e9085
3. Vrieze A, Holleman F, Zoetendal EG, de Vos WM, Hoekstra JB, Nieuwdorp M (2010) The environment within: how gut microbiota may influence metabolism and body composition. Diabetologia 53(4):606–613
4. Creely SJ, McTernan PG, Kusminski CM, Fisher FM, Da Silva NF, Khanolkar M, Evans M, Harte AL, Kumar S (2007) Lipopolysaccharide activates an innate immune system response in human adipose tissue in obesity and type 2 diabetes. Am J Physiol Endocrinol Metab 292(3):E740–E747
5. Remely M, Aumueller E, Jahn D, Hippe B, Brath H, Haslberger AG (2014) Microbiota and epigenetic regulation of inflammatory mediators in type 2 diabetes and obesity. Benef Microbes 5(1):33–43

6. Remely M, Aumueller E, Merold C, Dworzak S, Hippe B, Zanner J, Pointner A, Brath H, Haslberger AG (2013) Effects of short chain fatty acid producing bacteria on epigenetic regulation of FFAR3 in type 2 diabetes and obesity. Gene 537(1):85–92

7. Canani RB, Costanzo MD, Leone L, Bedogni G, Brambilla P, Cianfarani S, Nobili V, Pietrobelli A, Agostoni C (2011) Epigenetic mechanisms elicited by nutrition in early life. Nutr Res Rev 24(2):198–205

8. Dahaliwal A (2013) DNA extraction and purification. Mater Methods 3(191)

9. Kotorashvili A, Ramnauth A, Liu C, Lin J, Ye K, Kim R, Hazan R, Rohan T, Fineberg S, Loudig O (2012) Effective DNA/RNA co-extraction for analysis of microRNAs, mRNAs, and genomic DNA from formalin-fixed paraffin-embedded specimens. PLoS One 7(4), e34683

10. Wilfinger WW, Mackey K, Chomczynski P (1997) Effect of pH and ionic strength on the spectrophotometric assessment of nucleic acid purity. Biotechniques 22(3):474–476, 478-81

11. Muyzer G, de Waal EC, Uitterlinden AG (1993) Profiling of complex microbial populations by denaturing gradient gel electrophoresis analysis of polymerase chain reaction-amplified genes coding for 16S rRNA. Appl Environ Microbiol 59(3):695–700

12. Neefs JM, Van de Peer Y, De Rijk P, Goris A, De Wachter R (1991) Compilation of small ribosomal subunit RNA sequences. Nucleic Acids Res 19(Suppl):1987–2015

13. Muyzer G, Smalla K (1998) Application of denaturing gradient gel electrophoresis (DGGE) and temperature gradient gel electrophoresis (TGGE) in microbial ecology. Antonie Van Leeuwenhoek 73(1):127–141

14. Beutler E, Gelbart T, Kuhl W (1990) Interference of heparin with the polymerase chain reaction. Biotechniques 9(2):166

15. Willems M, Moshage H, Nevens F, Fevery J, Yap SH (1993) Plasma collected from heparinized blood is not suitable for HCV-RNA detection by conventional RT-PCR assay. J Virol Methods 42(1):127–130

16. (1993) Recommendations of the International Council for Standardization in Haematology for Ethylenediaminetetraacetic Acid Anticoagulation of Blood for Blood Cell Counting and Sizing. International Council for Standardization in Haematology: Expert Panel on Cytometry. Am J Clin Pathol 100(4):371–372

17. Raabe BM, Artwohl JE, Purcell JE, Lovaglio J, Fortman JD (2011) Effects of weekly blood collection in C57BL/6 mice. J Am Assoc Lab Anim Sci 50(5):680–685

18. Bustin SA (2000) Absolute quantification of mRNA using real-time reverse transcription polymerase chain reaction assays. J Mol Endocrinol 25(2):169–193

19. Griffiths-Jones S (2006) miRBase: the microRNA sequence database. Methods Mol Biol 342:129–138

20. Bui TV, Mendell JT (2010) Myc: maestro of MicroRNAs. Genes Cancer 1(6):568–575

21. Langevin SM, Stone RA, Bunker CH, Grandis JR, Sobol RW, Taioli E (2010) MicroRNA-137 promoter methylation in oral rinses from patients with squamous cell carcinoma of the head and neck is associated with gender and body mass index. Carcinogenesis 31(5):864–870

22. Langevin SM, Stone RA, Bunker CH, Lyons-Weiler MA, LaFramboise WA, Kelly L, Seethala RR, Grandis JR, Sobol RW, Taioli E (2011) MicroRNA-137 promoter methylation is associated with poorer overall survival in patients with squamous cell carcinoma of the head and neck. Cancer 117(7): 1454–1462

23. Egger G, Wielscher M, Pulverer W, Kriegner A, Weinhausel A (2012) DNA methylation testing and marker validation using PCR: diagnostic applications. Expert Rev Mol Diagn 12(1):75–92

24. Noehammer C, Pulverer W, Hassler MR, Hofner M, Wielscher M, Vierlinger K, Liloglou T, McCarthy D, Jensen TJ, Nygren A, Gohlke H, Trooskens G, Braspenning M, Van Criekinge W, Egger G, Weinhaeusel A (2014) Strategies for validation and testing of DNA methylation biomarkers. Epigenomics 6(6):603–622

25. Pulverer W, Hofner M, Preusser M, Dirnberger E, Hainfellner JA, Weinhaeusel A (2014) A simple quantitative diagnostic alternative for MGMT DNA-methylation testing on RCL2 fixed paraffin embedded tumors using restriction coupled qPCR. Clin Neuropathol 33(1):50–60

26. Morris T, Lowe R (2012) Report on the Infinium 450 k methylation array analysis workshop: April 20, 2012 UCL, London, UK. Epigenetics 7(8):961–962

27. Fortin JP, Fertig E, Hansen K (2014) shinyMethyl: interactive quality control of Illumina 450k DNA methylation arrays in R. F1000Res 3:175

28. Fortin JP, Labbe A, Lemire M, Zanke BW, Hudson TJ, Fertig EJ, Greenwood CM,

Hansen KD (2014) Functional normalization of 450 k methylation array data improves replication in large cancer studies. Genome Biol 15(11):503

29. Martens JH, Stunnenberg HG (2013) BLUEPRINT: mapping human blood cell epigenomes. Haematologica 98(10):1487–1489

30. Martens JH, Stunnenberg HG, Logie C (2011) The decade of the epigenomes? Genes Cancer 2(6):680–687

31. Ptitsyn AA, Weil MM, Thamm DH (2008) Systems biology approach to identification of biomarkers for metastatic progression in cancer. BMC Bioinformatics 9(Suppl 9):S8

Chapter 9

Optical Microscopy and Spectroscopy for Epigenetic Modifications in Single Living Cells

Yi Cui and Joseph Irudayaraj

Abstract

Optical imaging with high spatiotemporal resolution and analytical accuracy is becoming the mainstay of tools capable of deciphering molecular dynamics and activities in single living cells. Over the past decades, information obtained by optical imaging has greatly enriched and reshaped our knowledge of biology and medicine. Investigating epigenetic modifications by optical microscopy and spectroscopy is expected to be the wave of the future or might even become the norm to complement biomedical practice. Independent of classical genetic mechanisms, epigenetics has recently drawn substantial attention due to its extensive involvement in physiological and pathological processes, as well as its reversibility. In order to understand the real-time behaviors of epigenetic regulation, nanoscale inspection at the sub-second timescale is imperative. In this chapter we discuss the basics of state-of-the-art optical methods for life science research and their potential applications in imaging live-cell epigenetics. Moreover, with established experience in single-molecule detection, we provide practical guidance on how to choose and adapt optical instrumentations for different applications. Last, recent advancements and representative examples in sensing live-cell epigenetics are reviewed.

Key words Live-cell imaging, Single-molecule detection, Phototoxicity, Spatiotemporal resolution, Super-resolution microscopy, Light-sheet microscopy, FCS, FRAP, FRET, DNA methylation, Histone modification, Chromatin dynamics

1 Complexity of Probing Epigenetic Modifications in Single Living Cells

To capture epigenetic events in living cells, both at the spatial and temporal resolution the microscopy system should meet the scale of the ongoing cellular and molecular activities [1]. Spatially, the intracellular environment is extremely crowded. Given a human cell with an average volume of ~1 pL, three billion DNA base pairs (about 2 m if fully stretched) are compacted in its nucleus within a diameter of 10–15 μm. DNA methylation, occurring on cytosine, is one of the predominant epigenetic modifications and constitutes ~1% of human genome, which could create a fairly high in situ density of methylated cytosine (5mC) at specific

Barbara Stefanska and David J. MacEwan (eds.), *Epigenetics and Gene Expression in Cancer, Inflammatory and Immune Diseases*, Methods in Pharmacology and Toxicology, DOI 10.1007/978-1-4939-6743-8_9, © Springer Science+Business Media LLC 2017

Table 1
Timescale of biological activities in living cells

Timescale	Hours	Minutes	Seconds	Milliseconds	Microseconds
Cellular activities	Cell cycle progression; cell migration; differentiation; development	Endocytosis; exocytosis; transport; DNA damage repair; apoptosis	Biochemical metabolism; signaling; nucleosome assembly	Single-molecule diffusion; DNA replication; RNA transcription; protein translation	Molecular rotation and conformation change; enzymatic catalysis
	Phenotypic epigenetics		Molecular epigenetics		

regions, e.g., silenced gene promoters and heterochromatin sites. In another aspect, the genome-wide distribution of 5mC is heterogeneous and depends on the cell state, which comprises of another layer of complexity for time-course analysis in intact cells. Histone, as one of the most abundant protein species in eukaryotes, not only participates to form millions of nucleosomes but also harbors a wide spectrum of epigenetic modifications, such as methylation, acetylation and phosphorylation. These chemical marks, independent of DNA sequence, act in concert to fine-tune chromatin compaction and thus genetic events. In addition, hundreds of thousands of RNA (e.g., noncoding RNA) and protein factors implicated in epigenetic regulation further increase the intricacy of the epigenetic network, posing a significant challenge for live-cell monitoring.

For live-cell experiments, considerable emphasis should also be placed on the timescale of different cellular activities, especially those with a sub-second time span (see Table 1). In order for modern optical microscopy to capture and quantify the intracellular events, improvements in optics, electronics, and post-processing are all required.

2   Instrumentation of Modern Optical Microscopy

In the history of optical microscopy, the twentieth century has witnessed a plethora of revolutionary breakthroughs that rendered optical microscopy an irreplaceable part of life science research. The invention of fluorescence microscopes between 1911 and 1913 has initiated this technical leap and rapidly become the optimum for observing microorganisms and subcellular structures. Utilizing fluorescence-related principles, further developments of confocal microscopy (1961), total internal reflection fluorescence (TIRF) microscopy (1981), multi-photon microscopy (1990),

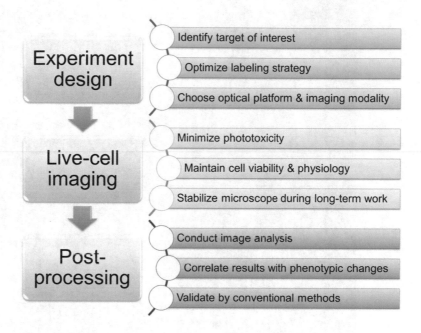

Fig. 1 Workflow for imaging epigenetic modifications in single living cells

light-sheet microscopy (1994), and super-resolution microscopy (1990s-present) have enormously improved the spatiotemporal limits of optical dissection. During this period, other microscopy modalities have also gained significant progress, such as label-free imaging with differential interference contrast (DIC) microscopy (1955) and stimulated Raman scattering (SRS) microscopy (1973). Given such a diversity of available tools, no "one-size-fits-all" platform exists for live-cell imaging. Herein a tentative general workflow for imaging epigenetic modifications in single living cells is outlined in Fig. 1 and the characteristics of microscopy methods described in this chapter are summarized in Table 2.

3 General Rules in Live-Cell Imaging

A single cell, especially of eukaryotic species, is composed of delicate organelles and active metabolism. Moreover, epigenetic mechanisms are vulnerable to a myriad of environmental variables, including temperature, pH, ion strength, viscosity, and osmolarity etc. Therefore, to image living cells, maintaining the cell viability and physiology is central to obtaining unambiguous information.

3.1 Phototoxicity

Even the light intensity required for imaging green fluorescent protein (GFP) would inevitably give rise to phototoxicity [2]. Hence, optimization for illumination and signal collection becomes critical to live-cell experiments. In regard to illumination, mono-

Table 2
Optical microscopy with quantitative capability for imaging living specimen

	Platforms	Illumination	Signal	Applications	Limitations
Transmitted light microscopy	DIC/phase-contrast/dark-field/polarized-light microscope	Wide-field illumination	Diffracted/refracted/scattered/polarized light	Imaging cell morphology, organelles and birefringence	Limited resolution and contrast
Confocal microscopy	Laser scanning confocal microscope	Laser, point scanning	Fluorescence	Biomolecule distribution and abundance	Low imaging speed and penetration
Multi-photon microscopy	Two-photon fluorescence/second-harmonic generation microscope	Transient high-flux of photons (e.g., from femtosecond pulsed laser)	Nonlinear anti-Stokes emission	Deep-tissue and live-cell imaging	Photodamage in focal plane and high cost of laser
Light-sheet microscopy	Selective plane illumination microscope	Thin-layer (1 μm) light from the sample side	Fluorescence	Developmental studies, deep-tissue imaging	Specialized instrumental alignment
TIRF microscopy	Objective-based (cis-) TIRF microscope	Evanescent wave illumination	Fluorescence	Single-molecule studies	Only access near-surface subjects
Super-resolution microscopy	STORM/PALM, SIM, STED	Highly modulated laser illumination	Fluorescence	Imaging finer cell structures	Special label or optics or mathematics required
Fluorescence lifetime imaging microscopy	Time-domain fluorescence lifetime imaging microscope	Ultrashort pulsed laser	Time-resolved fluorescence decay	FRET analysis, bio-sensing	Similar to confocal microscope
Raman imaging microscopy	SERS, CARS, SRS	(Near)infrared lasers	Raman scattering generated by vibration of chemical bond	Label-free imaging lipids or specific chemicals	Limited specificity

Table 3
The new generation of camera detectors

	Pros	Cons
ICCD	Single-photon sensitivity; picosecond-level gating speed	Need expensive image intensifier
EMCCD	High quantum efficiency; low noise with quick readout	Need extra cooling hardware
sCMOS	Large field of view; high dynamic range; fast frame rate	Low SNR under low-light condition

ICCD intensified CCD, *EMCCD* electron-multiplying CCD, *sCMOS* scientific CMOS

chromaticity, output stability and tunability are related to biocompatibility, for which laser and light-emitting diode (LED) are better choices than conventional fluorescent lamps. Also, far-red excitation (700–900 nm) is preferred for live-cell imaging due to minimal absorption and better penetration. In regard to signal collection, optical detectors with high quantum efficiency and signal-to-noise ratio (SNR) can significantly decrease the exposure time to prevent phototoxicity. On the basis of traditional charge-coupled device (CCD) and complementary metal-oxide-semiconductor (CMOS) cameras, the new generation of camera detectors is drastically advancing the versatility of live-cell imaging (see Table 3).

3.2 Environmental Factors

Other than providing a stable physicochemical environment, an imaging medium containing adequate carbohydrates, amino acids, vitamins, (deoxy)ribonuleosides, minerals, and other nutritional elements is often needed to maintain epigenetic homeostasis in time-lapse experiments. For instance, cells cultured in deficiency of folic acid will experience a radical reduction in DNA methylation. To image suspension cells or use light-sheet microscope, the position of specimen has to be precisely controlled and thus sample embedding with a transparent gel is required [3]. When applying any environmental changes, the cell state has to be reevaluated and normalized considering the epigenetic plasticity. Last but not least, during long-term imaging, the mechanical stability of the microscope has to be strictly controlled; otherwise some unexpected fluctuations (e.g., focus drift) could significantly undermine the data quality and lead to artifacts.

4   Epigenetic Information in Single Living Cells Enabled by Optical Microscopy

In eukaryote, the basic unit for epigenetic modifications to occur is nucleosome that contains a histone octamer core wrapped by 147 base pairs of DNA (Fig. 2). A multitude of chemical moieties, such as methyl- and acetyl- groups, can be enzymatically coupled to nucleosomal elements (e.g., CpG dinucleotide, amino acids at histone tail), then realizing the transcriptional regulation on relevant genes. The extremely small size of a nucleosome, which is approximately 10 nm, poses a daunting task for optical imaging methods to visualize and map a specific type of epigenetic mark in a single cell because of the existence of a physical barrier—diffraction limit. Due to the light diffraction, the spatial resolution of far-field optical microscopy is defined by Abbe's law: $d = \dfrac{\lambda}{2NA}$, which estimates the resolution limit for optical microscopes to be around 200 nm at best. In addition, nucleosomes are packed into chromatin fibers with tertiary structures and active motions. The technical imperfection constrained that the majority of biological analysis with traditional optical microscopy was only qualitative. With rapid development of technology, today more useful information can be extracted from an intact cell, even at the single nucleosome level. In this section, we will discuss live-cell imaging modalities that hold the potential to quantitatively decipher epigenetic modifications.

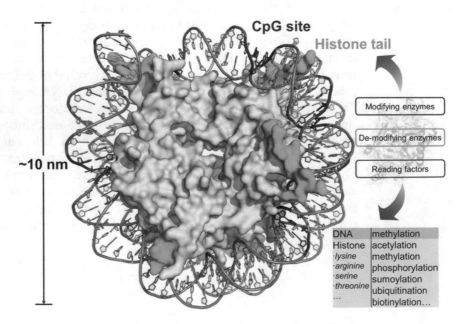

Fig. 2 Nucleosome serves as the basic unit and carrier for epigenetic modifications

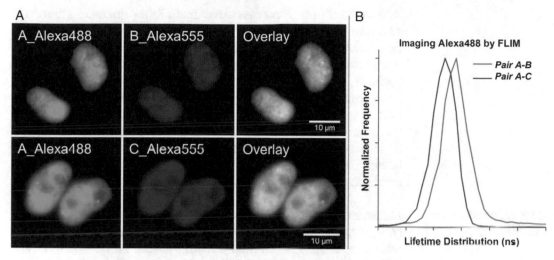

Fig. 3 FLIM-FRET is a superior approach to determine molecular interactions. (**a**) In conventional double-staining immunofluorescence assays, assessment of co-localization by color merging is not quantitative and subject to false positive results. Here, both A-B pair and A-C pair show certain extent of co-localization. (**b**) In FLIM, by comparing the fluorescence lifetimes of A_Alexa488 in the presence of different acceptors, it is clear that A-B pair has a closer association than A-C pair because C_Alexa555 evokes more reduction in the lifetime of A_Alexa488 due to FRET

4.1 Localization and Interaction

A major application of optical imaging is to assess the distribution pattern of the target molecules. As the time- and context-dependent epigenetic regulation involves the interplay between a myriad of editing and reading factors, high-definition visualization can enhance our understanding of the epigenetic dynamics and interactions. Yet for most cellular biomolecules, the physical size is far below 200 nm so that experimental artifacts are inevitable when using conventional imaging methods to evaluate their localization or co-localization (Fig. 3a). Hence, the precision of optical imaging exclusively hinges on how we circumvent the diffraction limit to locate the natural position of target.

4.1.1 Super-Resolution Microscopy

Over the last two decades, diffraction-unlimited imaging with super-resolution microscopy has significantly advanced our understanding of the intracellular intricacies. Using photoswitchable fluorophores, it is possible to excite only a few fluorescent molecules per imaging frame. Then the peak position of each molecule can be estimated by post-processing with a point spread function (PSF). After thousands of frames, a peak localization plot can be constructed. This is the working principle for stochastic optical reconstruction microscopy (STORM) and photoactivated localization microscopy (PALM), which at present can realize a lateral resolution near 10 nm. Another group of super-resolution microscopes makes use of specialized illumination patterns to break the diffraction limit. Representative techniques include stimulated emission depletion (STED) microscopy and structured illumination microscopy (SIM). Admittedly, there is no perfect super-resolution imaging platform for all applications. Besides the tradeoff between the imaging resolution, sensitivity and speed, sometimes a super-resolution platform has extra prerequisites. For instance, STORM and PALM require repetitive exposure and protective mounting buffer; SIM relies on complicated algorithm and is artifact-prone; STED demands specialized optical alignment and labeling materials. In spite of some promising attempts, super-resolution microscopy still needs be more amenable to living cells.

4.1.2 Förster Resonance Energy Transfer (FRET)

Discovered by Theodor Förster in 1946, FRET is the physical process of nonradiative energy transfer between two fluorochromes with proper spectral overlap and dipole–dipole orientation. The FRET efficiency (E) depends on the distance (r) between the donor and the acceptor with an inverse 6th power law: $E = \dfrac{1}{1 + (R_0 / r)^{-6}}$. FRET mainly manifests within an inter-dipole distance of 1–6 nm, and can serve as a biophysical ruler to measure molecular association and reaction kinetics. Changes in the fluorescence intensity or lifetime could reflect the occurrence of FRET and be quantified with different methodologies including sensitized emission, acceptor photobleaching, and fluorescence lifetime imaging microscopy based-FRET (FLIM-FRET) as: $E = 1 - \dfrac{I_{DA}}{I_D} = 1 - \dfrac{\tau_{DA}}{\tau_D}$, where $IDA/\tau D$ and $ID/\tau D$ are the fluorescence intensities/lifetimes of the donor in the presence and absence of the acceptor, respectively. Considering the reliability of results, we recommend FLIM-FRET to be optimal for FRET analysis since fluorescence lifetime is a more robust measure and independent of fluorophore concentration and excitation power (Fig. 3b). Otherwise systematic corrections for excitation and emission cross talk/bleed-through (the acceptor excited directly by the light for the donor, or the emission of the donor leaked into the detection channel for the acceptor) needs to be performed for intensity-based FRET analysis.

4.1.3 Gene-Specific Epigenetic Profiling and 3D Imaging

Epigenetic modification is locus-specific and functions in a 3D space, though current imaging techniques mostly provide global and 2D information. For gene-specific detection, both the DNA sequence and its nearby epigenetic marks have to be tagged, which has been successfully achieved with in situ hybridization-proximity ligation assay (ISH-PLA) in fixed cells [4]. However, ISH-PLA method is not a practical option for live-cell imaging since at least three rounds of labeling needs to be introduced into cells. Simplifying the targeting strategy becomes the key to realize gene-specific epigenetic profiling in single living cells. As DNA sequence-recognition modules, such as zinc-finger nucleases (ZFNs), transcription activator-like effector nucleases (TALENs) and CRISPR/Cas system, are rapidly arising, they can be implemented to specify a gene locus with fluorescent tags as well [5, 6]. Then the adjacent epigenetic marks can be labeled with antibodies or other affinity molecules. Conventional fluorescence platforms such as epi-fluorescence and confocal microscopes can achieve some extent of 3D imaging, but suffer from either limited penetration depth or excessive photobleaching. In comparison, multi-photon microscope and light-sheet microscope are superior systems to image the entire thickness of a mammalian cell (tens of microns) and even to achieve video-rate recording.

4.2 Quantity and Stoichiometry

Strictly speaking, methodologies to absolutely quantify an epigenetic mark in living cells are lacking due to technical hurdles, though analytical quantification is possible in fixed cells with fluorescence microscopy. A primary problem is that free probes are difficult to be removed from living cells by regular washing. Thus relative quantification for the target is frequently conducted with radiometric (intensity-based) analysis. In this regard, standardized delivery of probes and statistical analysis with a large number of sampled cells are necessary. Nonetheless, accurate quantification is possible with some newest techniques in which the specific signal can be separated from the nonspecific background. For example, a FRET sensor or molecular beacon-based probe can be designed, from which the "true" signal is detected only when a target is recognized. An alternative way to identify different states of probes is by comparing their biophysical parameters with single-molecule tools.

4.2.1 Fluorescence Fluctuation Spectroscopy

First developed by Douglas Madge, Elliot Elson, and W.W. Webb in 1972, fluorescence correlation spectroscopy (FCS) takes advantage of the spontaneous intensity fluctuations caused by fluorophores moving in and out of a femtoliter-level volume to biophysically extract molecular concentration, diffusion rate, and reaction kinetics (Fig. 4a) [7]. Time-resolved fluorescence fluctuation serves as the base to generate an autocorrelation function: $G(\tau) = \dfrac{\delta F(t)\delta F(t+\tau)}{F(t)^2}$, which describes the similarity between the measured intensities (F) as a function of lag time (τ). The autocorrelation function can be converted to approximation of single-molecule properties: $G(\tau) = \dfrac{1}{N}\left(1+\dfrac{\tau}{\tau_D}\right)^{-1}\left(1+\dfrac{\tau}{\kappa^2\tau_D}\right)^{-1/2}$,

where N is the average number of fluorophores inside the detection volume, k is the ratio of lateral (w_0) to axial (z_0) radius of the detection volume, and τD is the characteristic diffusion time.

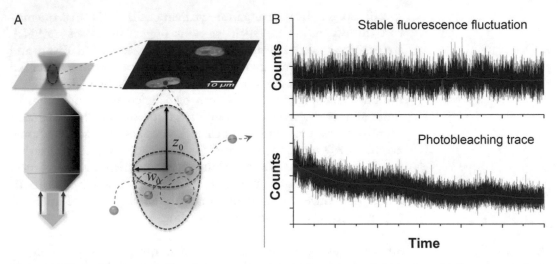

Fig. 4 (**a**) FCS enables the detection of single-molecule behaviors in subcellular regions. (**b**) Fluorescence trace with apparent photobleaching should not be used for downstream analysis

For more complex diffusing conditions, the autocorrelation function can be further expanded to higher-order models, such as multi-component diffusion, anomalous diffusion, and triplet state-corrected diffusion. By fitting with a proper model, the concentration of molecules with certain diffusivity can be calculated as: $C = N / V_{\text{eff}}$, where V_{eff} is the effective detection volume: $V_{\text{eff}} = \pi^{3/2} w_0^2 z_0$. Based on τD, the diffusion coefficient (D) of molecules can be calculated as: $D = w_0^2 / 4\tau_D$. The hydrodynamic size (R) of molecules could then be determined by using the Stokes–Einstein equation: $D = \dfrac{kT}{6\pi\eta R}$, where the molecular stoichiometry may be estimated as D is negatively proportional to R.

Stoichiometric heterogeneity and transition are implicated in numerous epigenetic events (e.g., oligomerization of DNA methyltransferase Dnmt3a, MBD-DNA binding stoichiometry, and catalytic modification of lysine monomethylation, dimethylation, trimethylation), but it is far from convenient to obtain this set of information from single living cells. FCS can be employed when molecular stoichiometry is strictly correlated with its hydrodynamic size. On the other hand, it is ubiquitous for stoichiometric alterations to be accompanied by conformational changes, which renders the relation between diffusion rate and molecular size not linear. Photon counting histogram (PCH) tackles this problem from another aspect—molecular brightness. In PCH, single-molecule brightness stems from an integration time-based photon histogram that can be fitted with a super-Poisson model. If the molecules of interest are uniformly labeled, their stoichiometry is

Table 4
Comparison between FRAP and FCS

	FRAP	FCS
Key parameter	Recovery of in situ fluorescence	Spontaneous intensity fluctuation
Optimal timescale	Milliseconds to seconds	Microseconds to milliseconds
Source of contrast	Mobile vs. immobile components	Fast-moving vs. slow-moving components
Concentration	Not available	Picomolar to nanomolar
Photodamage	High	Relatively low
Statistical significance	Depends on the size of ROI	Requires multiple measurements
Complexing ability	Not available	Possible with FCCS and FLCS

thereby proportional to brightness [8]. In theory, PCH and FCS are distinct approaches to interpret the fluorescence fluctuation profile but are mutually complementary [9, 10].

4.3 Dynamics and Kinetics

The ability of single-molecule spectroscopy and microscopy to monitor real-time information of intracellular dynamics is an unparalleled advantage. FCS, together with its derivatives such as fluorescence cross-correlation spectroscopy (FCCS) and fluorescence lifetime correlation spectroscopy (FLCS) are able to uncover a wide range of single-molecule characteristics. Besides FCS, fluorescence recovery after photobleaching (FRAP) and its variations is another set of imaging-based methods to study molecular biophysics at a timescale of sub-second (see Table 4) [1]. In FRAP, a defined area of the cell is photobleached with a high laser power and the recovery rate of in situ fluorescence is recorded; or a similar process is performed in fluorescence loss in photobleaching (FLIP) and inverse FRAP (iFRAP). The resulting intensity trace can be used to calculate diffusion behavior, association of molecules, and rate of transport in case a proportion of bleached fluorophores diffuse in space.

5   Representative Applications in Probing Real-Time Epigenetics

Advanced live-cell imaging, depending upon specialized expertise and expensive instruments, is still not commonplace in epigenetics research and faces continuous emerging challenges. Encouragingly, the cumulative findings by novel microscopic techniques have indeed extended our vision towards epigenetic mechanisms. In this section we introduce the most recent applications in probing single-cell epigenetics, and in parallel we provide some practical advice for several single-molecule tools.

5.1 DNA Methylation

First discovered by Treat Johnson and Robert Coghill in 1925, the 5-carbon in the pyrimidine ring of cytosine can be enzymatically methylated by Dnmt with the S-adenosyl methionine (SAM) as the methyl-donor. Once heavily methylated, the originally active chromatin becomes compacted and inaccessible to the transcription initiation complex, thus suppressing or silencing related genes. The status of DNA methylation substantively dictates the specific stage and the extent at which genes should be expressed. Hence, the regulatory machinery for cytosine methylation needs to be under rigorous control so that biological processes can proceed in an orderly manner. Conventional methods for evaluating DNA methylation, such as liquid chromatography tandem mass spectrometry (LC-MS/MS) and bisulfite sequencing, only obtain static observations from a population of cells, yet overlooking the cellular heterogeneity and intermediate dynamics. Live-cell imaging allows us to monitor DNA methylation in real time and directly correlate that with phenotypic alterations.

In order to label DNA methylation under its natural state, few options exist even if highly specific antibodies are available. The site of cytosine modification is deeply embedded in the DNA double helix and cannot be easily accessed by antibodies. Thus for immunostaining with 5mC antibodies, pretreatment of fixed cells with strong acid to expose the binding site is often required. Alternatively, utilizing the binding specificity between methyl-CpG-binding domain (MBD) proteins and DNA methylation provides an exclusive opportunity to label cytosine modifications. MBD is able to associate with methylated cytosine through hydrogen bond and cation-π interaction, which frequently assists in gene silencing (Fig. 5a).

The initial effort of adapting MBD as a sensor module was motivated by the need to visualize the pattern of DNA methylation in early embryogenesis. In traditional biochemical approaches, insufficient amount of samples that can be collected during pre-implantation development hindered a systematic analysis. However, this stage is extremely critical because the genome-wide DNA methylation is reestablished via drastic demethylation and gene imprinting. An EGFP-MBD-NLS fusion protein was then constructed at the mRNA level followed by microinjection into early oocytes or embryos [11]. By applying a long poly(A) sequence at the 3′-end and a cap structure at the 5′-end, the translation of this synthesized mRNA was greatly enhanced and the fluorescence signal can be detected after 3 h of injection. Thereafter time-lapse imaging was conducted to uncover the localization of methylated DNA in each stage of pre-implantation embryos [12]. Moreover, the observed phenomena or aberrancies regarding DNA methylation can be sequentially connected with developmental potencies since the living embryo can be transferred to host mothers after

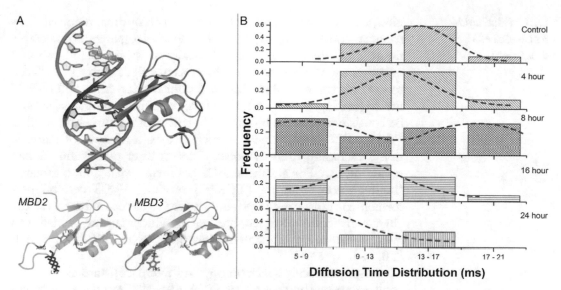

Fig. 5 (**a**) MBD belongs to a family of nuclear proteins in close relation to DNA methylation, but each MBD has its own binding property. In comparison with MBD2, MBD3 has a much lower in vivo binding affinity with 5mC due to the K30H/Y34F mutations, which makes it an ideal sensor for detection of DNA demethylation by FCS. (**b**) In hypoxia-induced active DNA demethylation, the mobility of MBD3 in living HeLa cells gradually increases (i.e., shortening of diffusion time), indicating the ongoing dissociation process

fluorescent imaging [13]. This technique has evidently revealed that incomplete reprogramming of DNA methylation gave birth to the low success rate of some assisted reproductive technologies including round spermatid injection (ROSI) and somatic cell nuclear transfer (SCNT).

Other than in embryogenesis, DNA methylation also experiences radical reconfiguration during oncogenesis, which features a global hypomethylation. Unlike other MBD homologues (i.e., MBD1, MBD2, and MeCP2), MBD3 has been suggested not to be a strong binding protein for 5mC due to amino acids mutation and incorporation into the Mi-2/NuRD complex. Nevertheless, the low binding affinity with methylation sites makes MBD3 an ideal candidate to monitor real-time DNA demethylation by single-molecule FCS (Fig. 5b). Ten-eleven-translocation (Tet) family proteins are the only enzymes responsible for active DNA demethylation in human and thought to promote cancerous hypomethylation. Overactive Tet-mediated DNA demethylation would force MBD3 to detach from its binding sites during cancer initiation and progression, which could generate more fast-moving MBD3 proteins and be detected by FCS in living cells. With this hypothesis, we have successfully recorded the detaching process of MBD3-GFP under the hypoxia-induced active DNA methylation [14].

First, the FCS methodology depends on an optimal range of fluorophore concentration (pM to nM level) to generate detectable fluorescence fluctuation. Second, ideally no photobleaching should occur during the collection of fluorescence signal. It is thus crucial to confirm the overall quality of the fluctuation trace before FCS fitting (see Fig. 4b). Third, the choice of a diffusion model should be consistent with the biological behavior of the target molecules. Fourth, FCS measurement is subjected to a number of parasitic noises including thermal noise, detector after pulse, and Raman scattering etc. For advanced FCS platforms with time-correlated single-photon counting (TCSPC) module, FLCS can be performed to statistically remove those noise elements based on the characteristic fluorescence lifetime of fluorophores, which can avoid unnecessary implementation of complex diffusion models [10, 15].

Single-molecule spectroscopy and microscopy are also potent tools to assess the motion of DNA methylation-related enzymes (i.e., Dnmt and Tet) whose proper association with target sites maintains the integrity of epigenome. CXXC zinc finger domains were thought to be critical for mammalian proteins involved in chromatin modification, especially with CpG sites. However, by characterizing the DNA binding activity with FRAP, it has been revealed that the contribution of CXXC domain to protein–DNA interaction is context-dependent [16]. The CXXC domain of Tet1 shows no in vitro binding affinity with DNA and thus is dispensable for the in vivo catalytic function. In contrast, the CXXC domain of Dnmt1 preferably interacts with unmethylated DNA substrates, though it is not the essential part for the in vivo methylating reaction either [16]. Further, live-cell FRAP has been applied to profile the cell cycle-dependent loading model of Dnmt1 onto chromatin, and suggested a PCNA-binding-domain-dependent (fast) loading in early S-phase as well as a targeting-sequence-domain-dependent (slow) loading in late S-phase [17]. Regarding the behavioral mode of Dnmt1 in DNA maintenance methylation, with a set of single-molecule fluorescence tools we have also identified a cell cycle-dependent co-operation between MBD3 and Dnmt1 to merit DNA methylation homeostasis in single living cells, which indicated a sophisticated network involved in epigenetic inheritance [10]. And by quantifying the free and bound forms of Tet1-catalytic domain with live-cell FCS, we have recently discovered that Tet enzymes might have a binding preference to hemi-methylated CpG and that contributed to an increased 5-hydroxymethylation (5hmC) in Decitabine-treated leukemia cells [18]. Altogether, these discoveries, impossible with conventional methods, will foster new perspectives for future biomedical research.

5.2 Histone Modification

FRET-based sensors for histone modifications have been first designed to monitor the real-time kinetics of modifying and de-modifying reactions at important positions [19, 20]. This group of tandem fusion probes usually contains five subunits: a substrate domain (histone residues), a flexible linker, a recognition module (varies based on the modification), and a pair of FRET fluorophores (e.g., CFP-YFP). Upon the addition or removal of a specific mark on the substrate, the probe would experience a conformational change to influence the FRET efficiency between the donor and the acceptor. For instance, by linking a chromodomain peptide with a fragment of histone H3 containing lysine K9 and K27, FRET signals can be detected in the presence of histone methyltransferases, both in vitro and in living cells [19]. With similar design, phosphorylation of histone H3 serine S28 can be sensed when replacing the chromodomain with a phosphoserine binding domain from the 14-3-3τ protein [20]. By monitoring the FRET intensity, the reversibility and fluctuation of histone post-translational modifications under different conditions have been quantitatively demonstrated. However, this first generation of FRET probes lacked of a full-length histone substrate and could not reflect the level of modifications in natural chromatin, which inspired the development of the chromatin-targeted probes. Termed as Histac, the new probe design included a full-length Histone H4 and the bromodomain of BRDT, for visualizing the dynamic changes of histone H4 K5/8 acetylation [21]. The successful implementation of Histac prompted the development of probes targeting other acetylation sites. The expansion of Histac toolkit enabled a comparison of the acetylation state at different positions in response to the same stimuli. For example, it has been found that the acetylation of H4K5 and K8 experienced a transient decrease during mitosis while the acetylation of H4K12 was kept constant throughout the whole cell cycle [22]. This is consistent with a relevant biological phenomenon that H4K12 acetylation is important for the immediate activation of genes necessitated for the G1-phase progression. Another important application of these histone modification probes is for cancer drug discovery [23]. Histone deacetylase inhibitors (HDACi) are emerging as a promising class of agents against some cancer types. Yet their intracellular behaviors and efficacy window has remained elusive. Live-cell imaging with Histac probes appears to be a feasible way to further our understanding of the epigenetic pharmacology of HDACi.

5.2.1 Practical Advice for FRET Analysis

1. The spectral properties of the donor and acceptor have to be strictly matched: the emission spectrum of the donor and the absorption spectrum of the acceptor should have a substantial overlap, whereas the emission spectrum of the acceptor should be distant from that of the donor to prevent bleed-through. In addition, it is beneficial to employ a FRET pair with comparable brightness.

2. In intensity-based FRET analysis such as sensitized emission, an algorithm that corrects the excitation and emission cross talk needs to be applied since the majority of available FRET pairs, especially fluorescent proteins, have a broad spectrum. In comparison, FLIM-FRET is a superior substitute for precise calculation of FRET efficiency in which only the donor fluorescence needs to be collected. When choosing a donor for FLIM-FRET, fluorophores with too short lifetimes should be avoided (e.g., Alexa Fluor 555 with a lifetime of ~0.3 ns).

3. When designing a FRET probe, the size and conformation of it should be carefully considered since FRET mainly occurs within a distance of 10 nm. Most of biomolecules are measured by mass (M), which can be practically converted to an estimated radius (R) using the equation: $R = 0.066M^{1/3}$ [24]. The orientation alignment between the donor and the acceptor is often neglected in biological FRET applications. However, for a pair of perpendicularly aligned donor-acceptor, FRET will not occur even if they are in a close proximity. Hence, a weak FRET signal requires cautious interpretation when the molecular interaction is evident from other experiments.

4. Intramolecular FRET is more quantitative than intermolecular FRET. The FRET-based probes for histone modifications mentioned above are all based on intramolecular FRET. The conformation-dependent FRET design avoids issues of with variable fluorophore concentrations.

In contrast to DNA methylation, histone modifications are accessible to antibodies in living cells, which allows the epigenetic marks on endogenous histone to be visualized with fluorophore-tagged antibodies. By fusing the antigen binding fragment (Fab) of mouse IgG with Alexa dyes, the phosphorylation of H3S10 was first imaged with this strategy [25]. This group of Fab-based sensors could rapidly enter nucleus due to a much smaller size (~50 kDa) than IgG (~150 kDa) and have no significant cytotoxicity. From FRAP analysis, the average residence time of Fab at its recognition site is less than 1 min, making it possible to monitor the quick changes of histone modification levels. The phosphorylation of H3S10, mediated by Aurora B kinase, participates in the chromosome condensation and segregation [26]. Live-cell imaging with Fab-based sensors has revealed that the deregulated phosphorylation of H3S10 led to chromosome missegregation in aneuploid cancer cells, bringing about a new insight to cancer pathology. Subsequently, Fab-based sensors targeting other histone H3 lysine modifications—methylation and acetylation—have been developed and implemented in mouse pre-implantation embryos [27]. One technical concern left for Fab probes came from their limited lifetime because the directly loaded or injected sensors were gradually diluted upon cell division. The newest version of Fab sensor "mintbody," by coding the desired cDNA fragments into a plasmid vector, can be stably expressed in vivo after transfection and selection [28]. This improvement greatly facilitates long-term imaging and could serve as an effective tool for high-throughput screening of epigenetic drugs.

5.3 Chromatin Dynamics

Consequently, epigenetic modifications will manifest their impact on the physical properties of local chromatin to adjust gene expression. Without live-cell imaging, it is formidable to capture the natural state of chromatin with high resolutions. Advanced optical microscopy fills the gap for us to directly monitor chromatin compaction, accessibility, and single-nucleosome dynamics.

In general, chromatin is categorized as heterochromatin and euchromatin depending upon its compactness, which is regularly visualized with DNA dyes in fixed cells. By assaying human cells expressing histone H2B tagged to either EGFP or mCherry with FLIM-FRET, the local density of histone, and chromatin compactness, can be characterized by monitoring the FRET efficiency [29]. In interphase, chromatin displays a range of compaction according to the observed FRET efficiencies, whereas in anaphase B chromatin is more uniformly condensed. Treatment with HDACi trichostatin A (TSA) significantly decreased the chromatin compaction, supporting the correlation between histone acetylation and decompacted state of chromatin. The heterogeneous organization and rearrangement of chromatin have also been measured with super-resolution 3D PALM [30]. In this work the authors have quantitatively shown the fractal nature of chromatin organization by imaging the 3D distribution of photoactivatable GFP (PAGFP)-labeled H2B at nanoscale, and suggested a dynamically maintained nonequilibrium state of chromatin density in living cells. However, the acquisition by PALM or STORM typically takes seconds to minutes, not ideal for imaging fast changes of chromatin, whereas light-sheet microscope enables a video-rate 3D imaging with low phototoxicity as mentioned above. Utilizing light-sheet Bayesian microscopy, recently the dynamic changes of heterochromatin have been imaged at a spatial resolution of 50–60 nm and a temporal resolution of 2.3 s [31]. This powerful tool is expected to benefit a wide range of deep-cell imaging and real-time probing. Our lab has recently developed a paired-particle tracking method to quantify macroscale movements of native chromatin using PAGFP-H2B [32]. This can achieve real-time readout of chromatin mobility free of the interference from cellular movement, and can be easily performed with a standard fluorescence microscope. Even though chromatin in mitotic phase is densely compacted, it still has considerable accessibility, revealed by live-cell FCS [33, 34]. This accessibility is predominantly attributed to a confined Brownian motion of nucleosomes. Utilizing another variant of light-sheet microscopy—highly inclined and laminated optical sheet (HILO) microscopy, the local mobility of individual nucleosomes was determined to be around 50 nm per 30 ms [33]. All these novel findings have refreshed our understanding of chromatin to suggest future research directions to explore the underlying epigenetic mechanisms.

6   Future Prospects

Until today, our understanding of epigenetic regulation is primarily due to large-scale and end-point observations using an ensemble of cells. However, epigenetic modifications are highly heterogeneous and dynamic. Metazoan species, especially human beings, contains billions of variedly differentiated cells that play fundamental roles in various biological processes. Cells within the same tissue or organ, at a given time point might have distinct morphological properties and functional states that are substantially dictated by epigenetic modulations. Single-cell live-imaging offers tremendous opportunities to inspect subcellular components with unprecedented resolution and accuracy. Modern optical microscopy and spectroscopy are particularly advantageous in characterizing epigenetic variation and inheritance implicated in embryogenesis and diseases in that most phenotypic features stem from single individual cells. Moreover, the increasingly potent microscopic tools will not only advance basic research, but also hold the promise in clinical diagnostics. Yet current imaging platforms developed for single-cell epigenetics are technically constrained at the global detection level. We anticipate that the booming sequence-targeting strategies will be soon adapted into observation of locus-specific epigenetics in single living cells. We also envision a bright future for label-free imaging in epigenetics research. In conclusion, quantitative information obtained from advanced optical imaging will constitute the basis for manipulating and engineering single living cells at the epigenetic level in near future.

Acknowledgement

The authors gratefully acknowledge funding from the W.M. Keck Foundation, National Science Foundation (#1249315), and Purdue Center for Cancer Research Core grant NIH-NCI P30CA023168.

References

1. Cui Y, Irudayaraj J (2015) Inside single cells: quantitative analysis with advanced optics and nanomaterials. Wiley Interdiscip Rev Nanomed Nanobiotechnol 7:387–407

2. Magidson V, Khodjakov A (2013) Circumventing photodamage in live-cell microscopy. Method Cell Biol 114:545–560

3. Huisken J, Stainier DYR (2009) Selective plane illumination microscopy techniques in developmental biology. Development 136:1963–1975

4. Gomez D, Shankman LS, Nguyen AT, Owens GK (2013) Detection of histone modifications at specific gene loci in single cells in histological sections. Nat Methods 10:171–177

5. Miyanari Y, Ziegler-Birling C, Torres-Padilla ME (2013) Live visualization of chromatin dynamics with fluorescent TALEs. Nat Struct Mol Biol 20:1321–1324

6. Anton T, Bultmann S, Leonhardt H, Markaki Y (2014) Visualization of specific DNA sequences in living mouse embryonic stem cells with a programmable fluorescent CRISPR/Cas system. Nucleus 5:163–172

7. Magde D, Webb WW, Elson E (1972) Thermodynamic fluctuations in a reacting system—measurement by fluorescence correlation spectroscopy. Phys Rev Lett 29:705

8. Chen Y, Muller JD, So PT, Gratton E (1999) The photon counting histogram in fluorescence fluctuation spectroscopy. Biophys J 77:553–567

9. Chen J, Nag S, Vidi PA, Irudayaraj J (2011) Single molecule in vivo analysis of toll-like receptor 9 and CpG DNA interaction. Plos One 6, e17991

10. Cui Y, Irudayaraj J (2015) Dissecting the behavior and function of MBD3 in DNA methylation homeostasis by single-molecule spectroscopy and microscopy. Nucleic Acids Res 43:3046–3055

11. Yamagata K, Yamazaki T, Yamashita M, Hara Y, Ogonuki N, Ogura A (2005) Noninvasive visualization of molecular events in the mammalian zygote. Genesis 43:71–79

12. Yamazaki T, Yamagata K, Baba T (2007) Time-lapse and retrospective analysis of DNA methylation in mouse preimplantation embryos by live cell imaging. Dev Biol 304:409–419

13. Yamagata K (2008) Capturing epigenetic dynamics during pre-implantation development using live cell imaging. J Biochem 143:279–286

14. Cui Y, Cho IH, Chowdhury B, Irudayaraj J (2013) Real-time dynamics of methyl-CpG-binding domain protein 3 and its role in DNA demethylation by fluorescence correlation spectroscopy. Epigenetics 8:1089–1100

15. Kapusta P, Machan R, Benda A, Hof M (2012) Fluorescence lifetime correlation spectroscopy (FLCS): concepts, applications and outlook. Int J Mol Sci 13:12890–12910

16. Frauer C, Rottach A, Meilinger D, Bultmann S, Fellinger K, Hasenoder S, Wang MX, Qin WH, Soding J, Spada F, Leonhardt H (2011) Different binding properties and function of CXXC zinc finger domains in Dnmt1 and Tet1. Plos One 6

17. Schneider K, Fuchs C, Dobay A, Rottach A, Qin W, Wolf P, Alvarez-Castro JM, Nalaskowski MM, Kremmer E, Schmid V, Leonhardt H, Schermelleh L (2013) Dissection of cell cycle-dependent dynamics of Dnmt1 by FRAP and diffusion-coupled modeling. Nucleic Acids Res 41:4860–4876

18. Chowdhury B, McGovern A, Cui Y, Choudhury SR, Cho IH, Cooper B, Chevassut T, Lossie AC, Irudayaraj J (2015) The hypo-methylating agent Decitabine causes a paradoxical increase in 5-hydroxymethylcytosine in human leukemia cells. Sci Rep 5:9281

19. Lin CW, Jao CY, Ting AY (2004) Genetically encoded fluorescent reporters of histone methylation in living cells. J Am Chem Soc 126:5982–5983

20. Lin CW, Ting AY (2004) A genetically encoded fluorescent reporter of histone phosphorylation in living cells. Angew Chem Int Ed Engl 43:2940–2943

21. Sasaki K, Ito T, Nishino N, Khochbin S, Yoshida M (2009) Real-time imaging of histone H4 hyperacetylation in living cells. Proc Natl Acad Sci U S A 106:16257–16262

22. Ito T, Umehara T, Sasaki K, Nakamura Y, Nishino N, Terada T, Shirouzu M, Padmanabhan B, Yokoyama S, Ito A, Yoshida M (2011) Real-time imaging of histone H4K12-specific acetylation determines the modes of action of histone deacetylase and bromodomain inhibitors. Chem Biol 18:495–507

23. Sasaki K, Ito A, Yoshida M (2012) Development of live-cell imaging probes for monitoring histone modifications. Bioorg Med Chem 20:1887–1892

24. Erickson HP (2009) Size and shape of protein molecules at the nanometer level determined by sedimentation, gel filtration, and electron microscopy. Biol Proced Online 11:32–51

25. Hayashi-Takanaka Y, Yamagata K, Nozaki N, Kimura H (2009) Visualizing histone modifications in living cells: spatiotemporal dynamics of H3 phosphorylation during interphase. J Cell Biol 187:781–790

26. Johansen KM, Johansen J (2006) Regulation of chromatin structure by histone H3S10 phosphorylation. Chromosome Res 14:393–404

27. Hayashi-Takanaka Y, Yamagata K, Wakayama T, Stasevich TJ, Kainuma T, Tsurimoto T, Tachibana M, Shinkai Y, Kurumizaka H, Nozaki N, Kimura H (2011) Tracking epigenetic histone modifications in single cells using Fab-based live endogenous modification labeling. Nucleic Acids Res 39:6475–6488

28. Sato Y, Mukai M, Ueda J, Muraki M, Stasevich TJ, Horikoshi N, Kujirai T, Kita H, Kimura T, Hira S, Okada Y, Hayashi-Takanaka Y, Obuse C, Kurumizaka H, Kawahara A, Yamagata K, Nozaki N, Kimura H (2013) Genetically encoded system to track histone modification in vivo. Sci Rep 3:2436

29. Lleres D, James J, Swift S, Norman DG, Lamond AI (2009) Quantitative analysis of chromatin compaction in living cells using FLIM-FRET. J Cell Biol 187:481–496

30. Recamier V, Izeddin I, Bosanac L, Dahan M, Proux F, Darzacq X (2014) Single cell correlation fractal dimension of chromatin A framework to interpret 3D single molecule super-resolution. Nucleus 5:75–84

31. Hu YS, Zhu Q, Elkins K, Tse K, Li Y, Fitzpatrick JA, Verma IM, Cang H (2013) Light-sheet Bayesian microscopy enables deep-cell super-resolution imaging of heterochromatin in live human embryonic stem cells. Opt Nanoscopy 2:7

32. Liu J, Vidi PA, Lelievre SA, Irudayaraj JM (2015) Nanoscale histone localization in live cells reveals reduced chromatin mobility in response to DNA damage. J Cell Sci 128:599–604

33. Hihara S, Pack CG, Kaizu K, Tani T, Hanafusa T, Nozaki T, Takemoto S, Yoshimi T, Yokota H, Imamoto N, Sako Y, Kinjo M, Takahashi K, Nagai T, Maeshima K (2012) Local nucleosome dynamics facilitate chromatin accessibility in living mammalian cells. Cell Rep 2:1645–1656

34. Nozaki T, Kaizu K, Pack CG, Tamura S, Tani T, Hihara S, Nagai T, Takahashi K, Maeshima K (2013) Flexible and dynamic nucleosome fiber in living mammalian cells. Nucleus 4:349–356

Chapter 10

MicroRNAs in Therapy and Toxicity

David J. MacEwan, Niraj M. Shah, and Daniel J. Antoine

Abstract

Identification of clinically important microRNAs (miRNAs) has developed over the last few years, and has become increasingly important in testing the role of miRNAs in healthy and diseased tissue states. Here we discuss the protocols of use in the laboratory for testing such roles of miRNAs in drug therapy and toxicity. Moreover, we describe the protocols necessary in a step-by-step practical guide to identify miRNA species, as well as the in vitro use of miRNA-modulating agents, to test the role of miRNAs in clinically important samples.

Key words AKI, Drug-induced acute kidney injury, AML, Acute myeloid leukemia, ARE, Antioxidant response element, DILI, Drug-induced liver injury, HMGB1, High mobility group box-1, KIM-1, Kidney injury molecule 1, miRNAs, microRNAs, NRF2, Nuclear factor (erythroid-derived 2)-like 2

1 Introduction

1.1 Role of miRNAs

MicroRNAs were first discovered just over 20 years ago, and since that time their importance in the regulation of normal gene transcription has developed exponentially. The function of miRNA is now considered crucial in most cellular processes to allow subtle modulation of all regulatory signalling within our cells. The majority of miRNA are indeed involved in a more fine-tuning of the processes involved in normal cellular function, with miRNAs acting to broadly repress a number of targets within a certain biochemical pathway or intracellular network [1]. Studies in evolutionarily early species including *C. Elegans* have shown with the systematic knockouts of miRNAs, they display some important regulatory role with much redundancy developed within the species. Although their effects are more limited, there still exists a small number that play a substantial role in their development [2]. There is increasing understanding as to the role that miRNAs definitely play in the regulation of gene transcription activities that underlie diseased states. As such, there is an increasing comprehension of the importance that miRNAs play in a wide variety of diseases from cancer through to long-term immune disorders and even in neurological disorders.

Barbara Stefanska and David J. MacEwan (eds.), *Epigenetics and Gene Expression in Cancer, Inflammatory and Immune Diseases*, Methods in Pharmacology and Toxicology, DOI 10.1007/978-1-4939-6743-8_10, © Springer Science+Business Media LLC 2017

There is also been found to have a role for miRNAs in pathological states that underlie drug-induced toxicities. As such, not only miRNAs modulate these diseased and damaged states, to play a function in modulating the cellular biochemistry to generate any negative phenotype, but their presence also may be indicative of such diseased or damaged states, and may well be suitable and practical biomarkers that will be a valuable prognostic tool in the clinic.

The miRNAs themselves are in fact noncoding RNA molecules that are synthesized in the genome and are often around approximately 19–24 nucleotides in length, typically 22-mers. These miRNAs are able themselves to bind and inhibit its target mRNA sequences through regular nucleotide-nucleotide pairing. MiRNAs can bind themselves, in a hairpin fashion, or complementary mRNA sequences to suppress the natural involvement of mRNA in translation promoted protein production. The biogenesis of miRNAs involves the RNA polymerase II transcription complex. Generated from specific genomic sequences that tend to flank regular coding gene sequences, miRNA gene sequences exist similar in nature to regular gene sequences but on a much smaller scale. It is not well understood how these miRNA gene sites are regulated themselves of what directs their activation and functions within cells. RNA polymerase II transcribes the miRNA into a long primary transcript that is known as a pri-miRNA. This pri-miRNA is then excised by an RNase III enzyme called Drosha to create the preliminary hairpin form known as pre-miRNA. Exportin-5 transports the pre-miRNA to the cytoplasm of the cell, where it is cleaved by the RNase endonuclease enzyme Dicer, which is essential for mammalian development [3]. This enzymic processing creates a short 19–24 mature miRNA transcript. In order to repress their mRNA targets, a mature miRNA associates with an RNA-induced silencing complex (RISC) via association and loading onto an argonaute (Ago) protein. Depending on the level of complementarity between the miRNA and its target mRNA sequence, further processing is possible, whereby RISC will either degrade or repress the mRNA transcript sequence itself, thereby blocking mRNA-directed translation and suppression of de novo protein production. It should be noted in mammalian cells the latter repressing process is predominantly the case rather than a potential degradation-type step [1].

1.2 miRNAs in Human Disease

As mentioned previously miRNAs are now clearly known to have a major role in the fine balance between healthy and diseased states. One such condition are a various chronic inflammatory and autoimmune conditions such as rheumatoid arthritis, lupus, and multiple sclerosis, where chronic pro-inflammatory cytokine generation extends the diseases and sustains the pathological tissue damage that is observed. One such example of the role here for miRNAs is the observation in peripheral blood mononuclear cells

(PBMC) from rheumatic patients of elevated miRNA species miR-203 [4]. The role of miR-203 included supporting the elevated expression of interleukin-6 and elevated nuclear factor-kB pro-inflammatory transcription factor levels, which drive tumor necrosis factor-α (TNF) cytokine production and associated damage. Indeed, one such study found that circulatory plasma from rheumatoid arthritic patients in early stage diseased state, show a miRNA signature that was indicative of their diseased state, which included miR-223 levels that tracked the progress of the diseases [5].

Cellular expression of miRNAs is universal, and these regulatory sequences are found within all cell types of the central nervous system. Long-term neurological diseases such as Alzheimer's disease and Parkinson's disease have recently found to contain interesting traces of critical roles for miRNAs. Cerebral spinal fluid and PBMCs from Alzheimer's patients were discovered to contain low levels of miR-29 prologues, which is known to lower expression of beta-secretase (BACE) 1 aspartate-directed protease that contributes to beta-amyloid protein accumulation and Alzheimer's pathogenesis [6], and may have a potentially protective effect [7]. In Parkinson's disease, postmortem brain tissue from patients that suffered from this debilitating condition, were found to have altered levels of miR-34 isoforms [8], but not miR-133 [9].

Human leukemias have recently been a rich source of miRNA regulation that needs to be overcome before treatment success rates improve. Acute myeloid leukemia (AML) is the deadliest form of leukemia where myeloid progenitor cells can rapidly progress tumorigenicity and virulence ultimately leading to accumulation of blasts cells within the bone marrow. AML is a heterogenous disease comprising a variety of genetic disorders, including molecular abnormalities commonly with mutations in nucleophosmin 1 (NPM1), CCAAT/enhancer binding protein-α (CEBPA), runt-related transcription factor 1 (RUNX1), or fms-related tyrosine kinase 3 (FLT3) internal tandem duplication (FLT3-ITD), or chromosomal abnormalities such as t(11q23) or t(8;21) [10]. miRNAs can be used to discriminate between different leukemia subtypes. One study used a genome-wide miRNA expression profile between acute lymphocytic leukemia (ALL) and AML, identifying 27 different miRNAs that displayed significant differential expression between disease subtypes, including miR-223 [11]. miRNA signatures were also identified from patients with cytogenetically normal AML (CN-AML), with 13 miRNA of lowered expression (miR-126, miR-203, miR-200c, miR-182, miR-204, miR-196b, miR-193, miR-191, miR-199a, miR-194, miR-183, miR-299, and miR-145) and 10 being upregulated (miR-10a, miR-10b, miR-26a, miR-30c, let-7a-2, miR-16-2, miR-21, miR-181b, miR368, and miR-192) [12]. It was uncovered that miRNA expression was a useful biomarker to help identify disease progression and prognosis, correlating high expression levels of miR-191 and miR-199a to poor prognosis in AML [12]. Another study in CN-AML identified miR-181a as another prognostic marker, being a good indicator for a milder prognosis and a reduced chance of relapse [13].

The miRNA miR-155 is a known oncomiR, defined as being is a miRNA that promotes carcinogenic mechanisms in cells, usually through repression of tumor suppressor genes. The converse of this is a tumor suppressor miRNA, which is anti-oncogenic in nature by inhibiting expression of cellular oncogenes [14]. In AML, miR-155 is processed from its parent gene miR155HG, which is located on chromosome 21 [15]. One study identified miR-155 upregulation in subtypes of AML such as acute myelomonocytic leukemia and acute monocytic leukemias of FAB subtypes M4 and M5, and ectopic overexpression in mice resulted in a myeloproliferative (pre-leukemic)-like disease [16]. PU.1 is an example of an AML tumor suppressor mutated in 7% of AML patients (primarily monocytic or undifferentiated leukemia) leading to inhibition of cellular differentiation processes [17]. As discussed later on, the miR-125 family exists as three homologues (miR-125 a, b, and c) originating from different chromosomes. The miR-125b form exists as two paralogs, miR-125b1 and miR-125b2, derived from a similar seed region but located on different chromosomes and therefore may be regulated independently of each other [18]. To date miR-125b remains the most well characterized member of the miR-125b family in leukemia. miR-125b-1 is overexpressed in AML cells particular of patients with a t(2:11)(p21:q23) translocation, showing a 90-fold increase expression levels [19]. Likewise, ectopic overexpression of miR-125b in mouse models leads them to developing leukemia, highlighting miR-125b's role as an oncomiR in blood cancers [20].

The transcription factor nuclear factor (erythroid-derived 2)-like 2 (NRF2) plays an important role in protecting cells from reactive oxygen species (ROS). We found in AML that NRF2 is constitutively activated and protects cells from front-line chemotherapeutic agents through its regulation of antioxidant genes [21]. Our work showed NRF2 positively regulates miR-125b1 and negatively regulates miR-29b1 in both AML. NRF2 regulation of miRNA was shown to increase resistance to chemotherapeutic drugs, and moreover, this chemotherapy-resistance was nullified when treated with a miR-125b antagomiR and/or a miR-29b mimic. As discussed later on also, antagomiRs and miR-mimics are short sequence RNAs that can be used as tools to inhibit or mimic cellular miR functions respectively [14, 22]. These antagomiRs and miR-mimic tools may be useful as pharmacological agents either to test the biology of a system of therapeutically influence a diseased cell's function.

1.3 miRNAs in Models of Drug-Induced Toxicity

To date, a major focus of attention directed toward the role of miRNAs in drug toxicity has centered on their role as biomarkers. Drug-induced toxicity not only has a major impact on the development of new medicines, as a leading cause of attrition, but also is a major reason for hospitalization and the safe use of otherwise efficacious drugs. Many organs represent toxicological targets for new or existing drugs but the liver represents on the systems that frequency represents an important safety issue and one that can range in severity from mild cell perturbation to fulminant organ failure and death. Therefore, herein we utilize the liver as a paradigm organ to address the potential role of miRNAs in drug-induced toxicity.

It has been widely cited that of the 10,000 documented human medicines, more than 1,000 are associated with liver injury [23]. The overall incidence of Drug-Induced Liver Injury (DILI) in the general population has been estimated to range from 10 to 15 cases per 100,000 patient years with the incidence of DILI resulting from an individual drug used in clinical practice ranging from 1 in 10,000 to 1 in 1,000,000 patients years [24, 25]. Although DILI accounts for <1 % of hospitalized patients presenting to hospital with jaundice [24, 26], it is an adverse event that most frequently results in regulatory action leading to black box warnings or removal of a drug from the market. In the clinic, DILI accounts for more than 50 % of acute liver failure cases, and improved detection of DILI before overt liver failure occurs has been the subject of intense investigation [23].

Drug attrition due to DILI occurs in all phases of the development pipeline, from preclinical testing to clinical trials to the marketplace. In cases where the frequency is high in either animal species or in humans, DILI is considered "intrinsic" in that it is assumed to result from direct hepatocellular damage [27]. However, another concerning manifestation of DILI, termed "idiosyncratic," occurs very rarely in susceptible individuals exposed to therapeutic doses [24]. The presentation of DILI (clinical and histological) can mimic most types of naturally occurring liver diseases. Idiosyncratic hepatocellular liver injury is generally the DILI of greatest concern because it can develop quickly and be life-threatening before the development of jaundice. Regardless of type, detection of DILI relies upon a small number of routine laboratory tests. However, there is a lack of specificity and sensitivity in currently utilized markers which leads to poor prediction of toxicity risk for individual patients or patient populations. The assessment of the potential for new chemical entities to elicit clinical hepatotoxicity is heavily dependent upon the histopathological evaluation of hepatotoxicity endpoints in preclinical species coupled with the quantitative assessment of circulating enzymes that are enriched in hepatic tissue [28, 29]. However, when clinical trials are performed, current preclinical testing regimens at best successfully correlate to clinical adverse hepatic events in about 50% of cases [30]. In addition, liver biopsies are not routinely taken from clinical trial subjects or patients with overt DILI, leading to incomplete assessment of the mechanisms of injury for a given drug. Therefore, there is a need to develop new and improved DILI biomarkers that can either confidently establish the diagnosis of liver injury early and to predict the course of patients (adapt, survive, develop liver failure).

The US National Institute of Health (NIH) defined a biomarker (for example an oligonucleotide, protein or metabolite) in 2001 as a characteristic that is objectively measured and evaluated as an indicator of normal biological process, a pathogenic process or a pharmacological response to a therapeutic intervention [31]. Biomarkers are classified by the US Food and Drug Administration (FDA) as exploratory, probable valid and known valid. A valid biomarker is further defined as a biomarker that is measured in an analytical test system with well-established performance characteristics and for which there is an established scientific framework or body of evidence that elucidates the physiological, toxicological, pharmacological or clinical significance of the test result [32]. Since then, recommendations have been set to avoid confusion that the term "validation" should refer to the technical characterization and documentation of methodological performances, and the term "qualification" refer to the evidentiary process of linking a biomarker to a clinical endpoint or biological process [33].

However, the development and clinical integration of potential hepatic biomarkers over the past 60 years has revealed only a limited number of candidates [29]. This concept is perhaps not so surprising given the fact that less focus has been placed on the science of drug safety and the rigorous guidelines we impose on the validation and biological qualification of a potential DILI biomarker [28, 33] compared to drug efficacy [34]. Furthermore, the delayed qualification and ultimate scientific acceptance of a potential DILI biomarker has been hindered by what has been previously thought of as the competing interest between the various stakeholders. Safety assessment within drug development has traditionally focused on reliable clinical-preclinical concordance. Low baseline variability, specificity and rapid analysis are sought after by clinicians and the ability to provide enhanced mechanistic understanding about toxicological processes is required by the academic community.

Many microRNA species show a high degree of organ specificity and cross-species conservation which makes them attractive candidates as translational safety biomarkers [35]. MicroRNA-122 (miR-122) represents 75% of the total hepatic miRNA content and exhibits exclusive hepatic expression. The majority of studies for DILI and miRNAs have been focused on the translational paradigm hepatotoxin, acetaminophen (APAP). MiR-122 has been shown to be a serum biomarker of APAP-induced ALI in mice, which was more sensitive with respect to dose and time than ALT [36]. The improved tissue-specificity of miR-122 versus ALT is supported by the observation that clinical ALT elevations associated with muscle injury are not accompanied by concomitant elevations in miR-122 [37]. MiR-122 has also been previously shown to serve as a clinical indicator of heparin-induced hepatocellular necrosis [38]. Moreover, as observed in mice, miR-122 is elevated in blood following APAP overdose in man and correlates strongly with ALT activity in patients with established acute liver injury. Furthermore miR-122 has been shown to represent a more sensitive biomarker of APAP hepatotoxicity in humans compared to currently measured clinical chemistry parameters [39, 40]. In these investigations, elevated miR-122 was observed in patients that present to hospital with normal liver function test values within the normal range but then later develop acute liver injury compared to those that did not develop acute liver injury following APAP overdose. Furthermore, lessons from healthy volunteer studies have also shown that increases in serum livers of miR-122 are associated with individuals that develop liver injury despite taking the therapeutic dose and that miR-122 rise at time points 24 h before ALT activity [41]. In these APAP overdose studies miR-122 correlated strongly with peak ALT levels [42]. The mechanism whereby miR-NAs can be released from "stressed" hepatocytes before the onset of toxicity are still under investigation and hold the potential to explain their added sensitivity for reporting liver injury compared to ALT. It has been recently demonstrated that in cultured primary human hepatocytes, cells can actively secrete miR-122 containing exosomes in the absence of overt toxicity [43]. Recent work may also show that NRF2 and miR-125b species may have additional critical roles in acute liver failure [44], suggesting roles for multiple miRs in drug toxicity models and organ damage settings.

Regarding the prognostic capability of miR-122, serum levels in APAP-acute liver injury patients who satisfied King's College Criteria (KCC) for liver transplantation, a specific measurement of the likely hood of needing a liver transplant to prevent death, were higher than those who did not satisfy KCC. However, this did not reach statistical significance, potentially due to small patient numbers [42]. Further prospective and longitudinal biomarker studies in acute liver injury patients will be required to determine whether miR-122 can provide added clinical prognostic value. The translational value of miR-122 as a sensitive circulating biomarker has also been demonstrated in an APAP overdose model in Zebrafish [45]. This represents an important observation for translational research and data interpretation given the increasing utility of this organism for earlier drug development studies. Despite, the advantages of miR-122, future efforts should be coordinated to developed cross laboratory validated methods for miRNA isolation and quantification as well as developing a consensus on normalization standards [46].

2 Materials

All standard laboratory reagents were used in these procedures. Sterile lab-ware was purchased from Gibco, Appleton-Woods or Starlabs. All other chemicals are of highest purity available and generally purchased from the Sigma Chemical Company. It is stressed that all buffers, chemicals, solvents, conditions, etc. are completely standard in generic laboratory conditions. The only exceptions to these are where it is necessary for the quality of the experimental data to be better than with our own buffers and chemicals, and as such, we would purchase the following premade kits. For miRNA extraction purposed, we utilize the miRVana miRNA extraction kit (Ambion). Qiagen miRNA reverse transcription kit (miRscript II RT Kit) allows efficient reverse transcription of miR species too. Our qPCR needs are served by the Lifecycler 480 SYBR Green Master Mix (Roche). The proprietary nature of Amaxa nucleofection technology ensures we use their Amaxa Nucleofactor Kit II for miRNA work—for all other purposes we find standard tRNA-containing media or even serum-free media useful media reagents for transfection or nucleofection.

3 Methods

3.1 Identifying miRNA Expression

1. Cell Culture—Cell lines were cultured according to standard sterile cell culture techniques in growth media containing serum, supplemented with essential L-glutamine amino acid and penicillin and streptomycin broad-spectrum antibiotics. Appropriate sterile-ware was used to contain and protect cell lines. Every effort was made to maintain protection of the cell lines from infection of any cross-contamination from rival cultures. The sterile flasks were incubated in standard humidified atmosphere at 37 °C, with a 95 %air/5 %CO_2 environment in order to equilibrate and buffer the media pH levels. Patient samples were treated similarly when sterile culturing was necessary.

2. RNA/miRNA extraction—Popular techniques for miRNA extraction include TRIzol and acid-phenol–chloroform extraction methods that retain miRNA species. We used the miR-Vana miRNA extraction kit (Ambion) which combines the two typical RNA extraction techniques: solid-phase and chemical extraction. Briefly, the cells are lysed in kit buffer, then straight acid-phenol–chloroform extraction is undertaken on the lysed cell extract in order to purify the RNA. The extract's total RNA levels (ie both mRNA and miRNA species) are then mixed with ethanol and placed onto a glass-fiber column to trap the RNA out of the sample. After a series of washes the

RNA can be eluted from the column. Extraction of small RNAs (i.e., miRNAs) follows a similar protocol, yet uses a lower concentration of ethanol, thereby allowing the small RNA to escape into the supernatant. After which the supernatant is further supplemented with ethanol and allowing the miRNA to become trapped when placed on a second glass-fiber column until elution.

3. RNA Spectral Purity—Spectrophotometer reading of the abundance and purity of both RNA and miRNA extracts are determined by standard procedures. We regularly use a NanoDrop spectrophotometer to assess abundance and purity. Some manufacturers do not recommend NanoDrop technology, but we have never encountered any issue.

4. Reverse Transcription—In order to reverse transcribe the mature miRNA we used a specific Qiagen miRNA reverse transcription kit (miRscript II RT Kit). Unlike their mRNA counterparts, miRNAs are not polyadenylated, and therefore, a poly(A) polymerase is used to add a poly(A) tail after which, the reverse transcription procedure can take place. In the miRscript II RT kit, both the polyadenylation, and the reverse transcription (using oligo(dt)) takes place simultaneously. The oligo(dt) primers also contain a 5′ universal tag, allowing quantitative PCR (qPCR) to be performed on the mature miRNA sequence.

5. qPCR Detection—Like mRNA, miRNA expression levels can be quantitatively analyzed using qPCR. The two main methods to perform qPCR are SYBR Green and Taqman. Our lab uses a SYBR green-based method using the Lifecycler 480 SYBR Green Master Mix (Roche) and qPCR was performed on a Lifecycler 480 fast real-time PCR machine (Roche). An important difference in analyzing miRNA from mRNA by qPCR is the use of primers. In a SYBR Green qPCR reaction, normally, mRNA targets are amplified by both sequence-specific primers for Forward and Reverse, and these are used to amplify that corresponding region of interest. However, in the case of a miRNA qPCR reaction, a miRNA-specific Forward primer is used in conjunction with a generic Universal Primer which replaces the Reverse primer. RNU6B (U6) and GAPDH are used as the internal reaction controls for miRNA and mRNA levels respectively. Melt curve analysis is used to analyze qPCR product specificity, and relative expression was analyzed using the ΔΔCT method.

3.2 miRNA Regulation

Distinguishing Individual miRNA Family Members—miRNAs often exist as both homologs and parologs. A miRNA homolog are two miRNA which comprise of the same seed region, but a different mature sequence (examples of which being miR-125a, b and c).

The seed region of a miRNA is a specific sequence of miRNA (usually around 2–7 nucleotides) that bind to its corresponding mRNA targets. Homologs will have the same seed sequences, but outside that, their mature sequences are different. On the other hand, miRNA paralogs are miRNAs which share the same mature sequence, but exist in different genomic location (for example miR-125b1 is located on chromosome 11 and miR-125b2 is located on chromosome 21). The mature sequences of both paralogs are the same, although originating from distinct sections of the genome. miRNAs can also be co-regulated alongside other miRNAs in miRNA clusters. For example, miR-125b1 exists in the vicinity of miR-100 and Let-7-a2, defining a local group, or miRNA cluster.

In order to identify which paralog was important to our study through qPCR methods, we found we were unable to use the mature miRNA sequence to distinguish between miR-125b1 and miR-125b2 [22]. Primers were therefore designed for the genomic flanking regions for both paralogs, as they exist in different genomic locations, and these flanking sequence will not be shared between the two paralogs. The paralog reverse transcription and qPCR steps are then carried out using the same method as mRNA qPCR, namely using a Forward and Reverse transcript-specific primer in the reaction, is used instead of use of a miRNA Universal Primer.

3.3 Manipulating miRNA Expression

1. AntagomiRs and miR-mimics—miRNA function can be manipulated using synthetic oligo nucleotides that act as miRNA mimics or miRNA blockers (termed as antagomiRs) [14]. Both miR-mimics and antagomiRs need to be introduced into the cell usually by standard transfection protocols. The miRNA mimics increase the functional levels of miRNA within cells. The miRNA antagomiRs block miRNA levels by binding to the mature miRNA form, thereby preventing the endogenous miRNA from repressing its target mRNA action. The design of miR-mimics and antagomiR has been carried out and tested by commercial companies, such as Ambion (Thermo Scientific) or Qiagen. These tested commercial miRs tend to be more effective than ones designed by ourselves. In our study we used these techniques to manipulate miRNA in AML. As with all hemopoietic cells, AML cells are notoriously hard to transfect. To that end, we used the Amaxa nucleofector machine for our miRNA transfection needs, utilizing the Amaxa Nucleofactor Kit II, that is more efficient at transfecting (or nucleofecting) MiR-mimic and antagomiR oligonucleotides into our hematopoietic cells.

2. Checking miR Effects—Commonly, the methods used to check whether your miRNA level manipulations have worked, you tend to leave the miRs to have their effect for around

24–72 h post-transfection. This is done in a variety of ways: to analyze the effects of miR manipulations on their target genes, qPCR is performed between 24 and 48 h post-transfection. For protein pathway regulation by miRs, Western blotting is usually performed 48–72 h post-transfection. Importantly, it is worth noting, that miRNA targets can be cell-type specific. As such, some cells may respond more efficiently than others to miR effects.

4 Notes

All standard laboratory reagents were used in these procedures. Sterile cell culturing, and molecular biological techniques we find give better results when fresh buffers are used for experiments. For example, freshly made SDS-PAGE gels and buffers offer superior quality separation compared to vastly more expensive pre-cast gels or buffers, that have been made up months beforehand. Exceptions of factory-made kits where quality is improved by their use include the miRVana miRNA extraction kit (Ambion), miRscript II miRNA reverse transcription kit (Qiagen), Lifecycler 480 SYBR Green Master Mix (Roche), and the Amaxa Nucleofactor Kit II for miRNA transfections. There are online tools such as www.mirbase.org who have already characterized miR and their effects, which we have found to be extremely helpful in the lab. It should also be noted for the main part, that miRNAs are modulators of cellular responses, not their driving forces. As such, do not expect large variations of target responses.

References

1. Garzon R, Marcucci G, Croce CM (2010) Targeting microRNAs in cancer: rationale, strategies and challenges. Nat Rev Drug Discov 9:775–789

2. Miska EA, Alvarez-Saavedra E, Abbott AL, Lau NC, Hellman AB, McGonagle SM, Bartel DP, Ambros VR, Horvitz HR (2007) Most Caenorhabditis elegans microRNAs are individually not essential for development or viability. PLoS Genet 3, e215

3. Bernstein E, Kim SY, Carmell MA, Murchison EP, Alcorn H, Li MZ, Mills AA, Elledge SJ, Anderson KV, Hannon GJ (2003) Dicer is essential for mouse development. Nat Genet 35:215–217

4. Stanczyk J, Ospelt C, Karouzakis E, Filer A, Raza K, Kolling C, Gay R, Buckley CD, Tak PP, Gay S, Kyburz D (2011) Altered expression of microRNA-203 in rheumatoid arthritis synovial fibroblasts and its role in fibroblast activation. Arthritis Rheum 63:373–381

5. Filkova M, Aradi B, Senolt L, Ospelt C, Vettori S, Mann H, Filer A, Raza K, Buckley CD, Snow M, Vencovsky J, Pavelka K, Michel BA, Gay RE, Gay S, Jungel A (2014) Association of circulating miR-223 and miR-16 with disease activity in patients with early rheumatoid arthritis. Ann Rheum Dis 73:1898–1904

6. Wang WX, Huang Q, Hu Y, Stromberg AJ, Nelson PT (2011) Patterns of microRNA expression in normal and early Alzheimer's disease human temporal cortex: white matter versus gray matter. Acta Neuropathol 121:193–205

7. Yang G, Song Y, Zhou X, Deng Y, Liu T, Weng G, Yu D, Pan S (2015) MicroRNA-29c targets beta-site amyloid precursor protein-cleaving enzyme 1 and has a neuroprotective

role in vitro and in vivo. Mol Med Rep 12:3081–3088

8. Minones-Moyano E, Porta S, Escaramis G, Rabionet R, Iraola S, Kagerbauer B, Espinosa-Parrilla Y, Ferrer I, Estivill X, Marti E (2011) MicroRNA profiling of Parkinson's disease brains identifies early downregulation of miR-34b/c which modulate mitochondrial function. Hum Mol Genet 20:3067–3078

9. de Mena L, Coto E, Cardo LF, Diaz M, Blazquez M, Ribacoba R, Salvador C, Pastor P, Samaranch L, Moris G, Menendez M, Corao AI, Alvarez V (2010) Analysis of the micro-RNA-133 and PITX3 genes in Parkinson's disease. Am J Med Genet B Neuropsychiatr Genet 153b:234–1239

10. Dohner K, Dohner H (2008) Molecular characterization of acute myeloid leukemia. Haematol-Hematol J 93:976–982

11. Mi SL, Lu J, Sun M, Li ZJ, Zhang H, Neilly MB, Wang Y, Qian ZJ, Jin J, Zhang YM, Bohlander SK, Le Beau MM, Larson RA, Golub TR, Rowley JD, Chen JJ (2007) MicroRNA expression signatures accurately discriminate acute lymphoblastic leukemia from acute myeloid leukemia. Proc Natl Acad Sci U S A 104:19971–19976

12. Garzon R, Volinia S, Liu CG, Fernandez-Cymering C, Palumbo T, Pichiorri F, Fabbri M, Coombes K, Alder H, Nakamura T, Flomenberg N, Marcucci G, Calin GA, Kornblau SM, Kantarjian H, Bloomfield CD, Andreeff M, Croce CM (2008) MicroRNA signatures associated with cytogenetics and prognosis in acute myeloid leukemia. Blood 111:3183–3189

13. Schwind S, Maharry K, Radmacher MD, Mrozek K, Holland KB, Margeson D, Whitman SP, Hickey C, Becker H, Metzeler KH, Paschka P, Baldus CD, Liu SJ, Garzon R, Powell BL, Kolitz JE, Carroll AJ, Caligiuri MA, Larson RA, Marcucci G, Bloomfield CD (2010) Prognostic significance of expression of a single microRNA, miR-181a, in cytogenetically normal acute myeloid leukemia: a cancer and leukemia group B study. J Clin Oncol 28:5257–5264

14. Shah NM, Rushworth SA, Murray MY, Bowles KM, MacEwan DJ (2013) Understanding the role of NRF2-regulated miRNAs in human malignancies. Oncotarget 4:1130–1142

15. Elton TS, Selemon H, Elton SM, Parinandi NL (2013) Regulation of the MIR155 host gene in physiological and pathological processes. Gene 532:1–12

16. O'Connell RM, Rao DS, Chaudhuri AA, Boldin MP, Taganov KD, Nicoll J, Paquette RL, Baltimore D (2008) Sustained expression of microRNA-155 in hematopoietic stem cells causes a myeloproliferative disorder. J Exp Med 205:585–594

17. Mueller BU, Pabst T, Osato M, Asou N, Johansen LM, Minden MD, Behre G, Hiddemann W, Ito Y, Tenen DG (2003) Heterozygous PU.1 mutations are associated with acute myeloid leukemia. Blood 101:2074

18. Shaham L, Binder V, Gefen N, Borkhardt A, Izraeli S (2012) MiR-125 in normal and malignant hematopoiesis. Leukemia 26:2011–2018

19. Bousquet M, Quelen C, Rosati R, Mansat-De Mas R, La Starza R, Bastard C, Lippert E, Talmant P, Lafage-Pochitaloff M, Leroux D, Gervais C, Viguie F, Lai JL, Terre C, Beverlo B, Sambani C, Hagemeijer A, Marynen P, Delsol G, Dastugue N, Mecucci C, Brousset P (2008) Myeloid cell differentiation arrest by miR-125b-1 in myelodysplasic syndrome and acute myeloid leukemia with the t(2;11)(p21;q23) translocation. J Exp Med 205:2499–2506

20. Bousquet M, Harris M, Zhou BY, Fleming MD, Lodish H (2010) MicroRNA Mir-125b causes leukemia. Blood 116:1299

21. Rushworth SA, Zaitseva L, Murray MY, Shah NM, Bowles KM, MacEwan DJ (2012) The high Nrf2 expression in human acute myeloid leukemia is driven by NF-kappa B and underlies its chemo-resistance. Blood 120:5188–5198

22. Shah NM, Zaitseva L, Bowles KM, MacEwan DJ, Rushworth SA (2015) NRF2-driven miR-125B1 and miR-29B1 transcriptional regulation controls a novel anti-apoptotic miRNA regulatory network for AML survival. Cell Death Differ 22:654–664

23. Lee WM (2003) Drug-induced hepatotoxicity. N Engl J Med 349:474–485

24. Sgro C, Clinard F, Ouazir K, Chanay H, Allard C, Guilleminet C, Lenoir C, Lemoine A, Hillon P (2002) Incidence of drug-induced hepatic injuries: a French population-based study. Hepatology 36:451–455

25. Meier Y, Cavallaro M, Roos M, Pauli-Magnus C, Folkers G, Meier PJ, Fattinger K (2005) Incidence of drug-induced liver injury in medical inpatients. Eur J Clin Pharmacol 61:135–143

26. Vuppalanchi R, Liangpunsakul S, Chalasani N (2007) Etiology of new-onset jaundice: how often is it caused by idiosyncratic drug-induced liver injury in the United States? Am J Gastroenterol 102:558–562, quiz 693

27. Corsini A, Ganey P, Ju C, Kaplowitz N, Pessayre D, Roth R, Watkins PB, Albassam M, Liu B, Stancic S, Suter L, Bortolini M (2012)

Current challenges and controversies in drug-induced liver injury. Drug Saf 35:1099–1117

28. Moggs J, Moulin P, Pognan F, Brees D, Leonard M, Busch S, Cordier A, Heard DJ, Kammuller M, Merz M, Bouchard P, Chibout SD (2012) Investigative safety science as a competitive advantage for pharma. Expert Opin Drug Metab Toxicol 8:1071–1082

29. Antoine DJ, Mercer AE, Williams DP, Park BK (2009) Mechanism-based bioanalysis and biomarkers for hepatic chemical stress. Xenobiotica 39:565–577

30. Olson H, Betton G, Robinson D, Thomas K, Monro A, Kolaja G, Lilly P, Sanders J, Sipes G, Bracken W, Dorato M, Van Deun K, Smith P, Berger B, Heller A (2000) Concordance of the toxicity of pharmaceuticals in humans and in animals. Regul Toxicol Pharmacol 32:56–67

31. Biomarkers Definitions Working G (2001) Biomarkers and surrogate endpoints: preferred definitions and conceptual framework. Clin Pharmacol Ther 69:89–95

32. Ratner M (2005) FDA pharmacogenomics guidance sends clear message to industry. Nat Rev Drug Discov 4:359

33. Matheis K, Laurie D, Andriamandroso C, Arber N, Badimon L, Benain X, Bendjama K, Clavier I, Colman P, Firat H, Goepfert J, Hall S, Joos T, Kraus S, Kretschmer A, Merz M, Padro T, Planatscher H, Rossi A, Schneiderhan-Marra N, Schuppe-Koistinen I, Thomann P, Vidal JM, Molac B (2011) A generic operational strategy to qualify translational safety biomarkers. Drug Discov Today 16:600–608

34. Watkins PB (2011) Drug safety sciences and the bottleneck in drug development. Clin Pharmacol Ther 89:788–790

35. Zen K, Zhang CY (2012) Circulating microRNAs: a novel class of biomarkers to diagnose and monitor human cancers. Med Res Rev 32:326–348

36. Wang K, Zhang S, Marzolf B, Troisch P, Brightman A, Hu Z, Hood LE, Galas DJ (2009) Circulating microRNAs, potential biomarkers for drug-induced liver injury. Proc Natl Acad Sci U S A 106:4402–4407

37. Zhang Y, Jia Y, Zheng R, Guo Y, Wang Y, Guo H, Fei M, Sun S (2010) Plasma microRNA-122 as a biomarker for viral-, alcohol-, and chemical-related hepatic diseases. Clin Chem 56:1830–1838

38. Harrill AH, Roach J, Fier I, Eaddy JS, Kurtz CL, Antoine DJ, Spencer DM, Kishimoto TK, Pisetsky DS, Park BK, Watkins PB (2012) The effects of heparins on the liver: application of mechanistic serum biomarkers in a randomized study in healthy volunteers. Clin Pharmacol Ther 92:214–220

39. Antoine DJ, Dear JW, Lewis PS, Platt V, Coyle J, Masson M, Thanacoody RH, Gray AJ, Webb DJ, Moggs JG, Bateman DN, Goldring CE, Park BK (2013) Mechanistic biomarkers provide early and sensitive detection of acetaminophen-induced acute liver injury at first presentation to hospital. Hepatology 58:777–787

40. Dear JW, Antoine DJ, Starkey-Lewis P, Goldring CE, Park BK (2013) Letter to the editor: early detection of paracetamol toxicity using circulating liver microRNA and markers of cell necrosis. Br J Clin Pharmacol. doi: 10.1111/bcp.12214

41. Thulin P, Nordahl G, Gry M, Yimer G, Aklillu E, Makonnen E, Aderaye G, Lindquist L, Mattsson CM, Ekblom B, Antoine DJ, Park BK, Linder S, Harrill AH, Watkins PB, Glinghammar B, Schuppe-Koistinen I (2014) Keratin-18 and microRNA-122 complement alanine aminotransferase as novel safety biomarkers for drug-induced liver injury in two human cohorts. Liver Int. 34:367–378

42. Starkey Lewis PJ, Dear J, Platt V, Simpson KJ, Craig DG, Antoine DJ, French NS, Dhaun N, Webb DJ, Costello EM, Neoptolemos JP, Moggs J, Goldring CE, Park BK (2011) Circulating microRNAs as potential markers of human drug-induced liver injury. Hepatology 54:1767–1776

43. Holman NS, Mosedale M, Wolf KK, LeCluyse EL, Watkins PB (2016) Subtoxic alterations in hepatocyte-derived exosomes: an early step in drug-induced liver injury? Toxicol Sci 151:365–375

44. Yang D, Yuan Q, Balakrishnan A, Bantel H, Klusmann JH, Manns MP, Ott M, Cantz T, Sharma AD (2016) MicroRNA-125b-5p mimic inhibits acute liver failure. Nat Commun 7:11916

45. Vliegenthart AD, Starkey Lewis P, Tucker CS, Del Pozo J, Rider S, Antoine DJ, Dubost V, Westphal M, Moulin P, Bailey MA, Moggs JG, Goldring CE, Park BK, Dear JW (2014) Retro-orbital blood acquisition facilitates circulating microRNA measurement in zebrafish with paracetamol hepatotoxicity. Zebrafish 11:219–226

46. Sharkey JW, Antoine DJ, Park BK (2012) Validation of the isolation and quantification of kidney enriched miRNAs for use as biomarkers. Biomarkers 17:231–239

Chapter 11

Genetics and Epigenetics of Multiple Sclerosis

Borut Peterlin, Ales Maver, Vidmar Lovro, and Luca Lovrečić

Abstract

Multiple sclerosis (MS), a chronic inflammatory neurodegenerative disease of the central nervous system (CNS), mainly affects young adults between 20 and 40 years of age and, therefore, presents an important health burden in the active population. Disease etiology is still largely unknown and different "omic" approaches, some of them available only in the last few years, are considered to be of great importance for deciphering the pathophysiology, progression and different subtypes of the disease. Combining results from exome sequencing, genome-wide association studies, transcriptome and epigenome levels, we gained insights into different levels of whole genome cell specific changes. The integratomic approach provides evidence for dysregulated JAK-STAT signaling pathway in MS, which is shown to be different in MS patients when compared to controls in all abovementioned different genome-wide approaches.

Key words Multiple sclerosis, GWAS, Transcriptomics, Epigenetics, Genetics

1 Introduction

Multiple sclerosis (MS) is a chronic inflammatory and neurodegenerative disease of the central nervous system (CNS) that mainly affects young adults between 20 and 40 years of age. In the course of the disease most patients develop a substantial disability, which creates an important burden for themselves, their families and society. The etiology of disease is still largely unknown; it is considered that multiple environmental and genetic factors contribute and interact in the pathogenesis of the disease. Epidemiological studies indicate that Epstein-Barr virus infections, tobacco smoking and lower sun exposure and vitamin D levels are risk factors for developing MS [1]. Furthermore, it seems that certain diseases like cancer, especially cervical, breast and digestive cancers, hypertension and stroke occur in patients with MS more frequently than in the general population [2]. On the other hand, familial clustering of the disease, determined importantly by genetic factors [3] has so far not led to an identification of high penetrant genetic variants as was the case in several other common neurological diseases

Barbara Stefanska and David J. MacEwan (eds.), *Epigenetics and Gene Expression in Cancer, Inflammatory and Immune Diseases*, Methods in Pharmacology and Toxicology, DOI 10.1007/978-1-4939-6743-8_11, © Springer Science+Business Media LLC 2017

including Alzheimer's disease, Parkinson's disease and amyotrophic lateral sclerosis. Current evidence suggests a polygenic model with a multiplicative model of one locus of moderate effect with many loci of small effect [4]. The understanding of interactions among environmental and genetic factors is still in its infancy. Nevertheless, there is some evidence for the interaction among environmental and genetic factors related to vitamin D biology including association among genetic variability in vitamin D receptor gene—VDR, vitamin D activating enzyme—CYP27B1 and vitamin D breakdown enzyme CYP24A1 and vitamin D [5]. Despite a considerable progress in deciphering mechanisms of MS, we do not know what causes MS and new hypothesis are needed for better treatment and prevention of the disease. Hypothesis free approaches like genome wide association studies (GWAS), transcriptomics and epigenomics as well as their integration might shed new light on the etiology and pathogenesis of MS. In this chapter we review the current impact of mentioned omic approaches on understanding MS.

2   Genome-Wide Genetic Surveys in Multiple Sclerosis

Considering the large body of epidemiological evidence for the role of genetic factors in the development of multiple sclerosis, a number of genetic studies have been performed aiming to delineate the contribution inherited variation in the risk of MS development. While the contribution of human leukocyte antigen (HLA) region has been repeatedly associated with the risk of MS development, a considerable proportion of MS heritability still could not be explained by variation on 6p21 chromosome [6, 7]. For this reason, a number of studies have continued the search of non-HLA loci, associated with MS risk with the search greatly accelerated by the development of new technologies for high-throughput microarray-based determination of genetic variation.

Initial studies have focused on using identifying regions linked with MS susceptibility with microsatellite linkage scans in multiplex families, but these have only been able to replicate the association within the 6p21 region [8]. The linkage studies were primarily limited to analyzing families with multiple numbers of affected individuals, which significantly limited the number of individuals that could be included in the genetic analyses and thus limited the power to detect further contributory genetic loci. Discovery and characterization of a large number of single nucleotide polymorphisms (SNPs) in the human genome and the advances in technologies for high-throughput interrogation of SNP variants made it possible to carry out studies testing for association of markers across the whole human genome with susceptibility to human disease (genome-wide association studies).

An initial GWAS in multiple sclerosis was performed in 2007 by the International Multiple Sclerosis Genetics Consortium (IMSGC), typing 334,923 single nucleotide polymorphisms (SNPs) in 931 trios with an affected child [9]. In addition to HLA loci, this study already had sufficient power to detect association in two non-HLA loci, including IL2RA and IL7R genes. Both identified genes have clearly established functions in the development and regulation of immune response with IL7R being part of a crucial and nonredundant immune pathway for proliferation and survival of T and B lymphocytes and IL2RA-associated variants are now known to regulate the propensity of naïve Th cells into memory Th cells [10].

Following the initial GWAS, a number of other teams followed-up to bring the number of such scans to 14 by year 2011 [8] (Table 1), providing convincing evidence for association of multiple non-HLA genes with susceptibility to MS. The sensitivity of genome-wide association studies is directly related to the number of samples screened, meaning that more recent and larger studies involving over 1000 participants enabled detection of non-HLA risk variants with minor risk effects. The largest GWAS to date was performed in 2011, building upon collaboration between IMSGC and Wellcome Trust Case Control Consortium (WTCCC2), which included 9772 patients and a comparable number of 17,376 controls in the study. An increase in the size of the studied group also greatly increased the power to detect genetic loci with minor effects, expanding the number of associated non-HLA loci to 57 candidate regions [11]. Top genome-wide association hits overwhelmingly map the regions of genes involved in biological processes of lymphocyte activation and T-cell activation, which aligns to the hypothesis of inflammatory processes in multiple sclerosis being caused by the appearance of auto-reactive T-lymphocytes, crossing the blood–brain barrier and causing demyelination in the central nervous system.

Although results from various association studies overlap only partially, there appears to be a somewhat clear convergence of detected hits, especially among the more recent studies with larger sample sizes included in the survey. A number of non-HLA genes have consistently been replicated in different studies and across various populations, including IL2RA and CD58, which have been reported in five separate studies, according to NHGRI catalog of GWAS (Fig. 1). Furthermore, the Immunochip analysis of over 150,000 SNPs implicated in MS and other related immune disorders was performed as a means of large scale validation of genetic loci, identified in GWA studies. In a large cohort of 14,498 cases and 24,091 controls these new results convincingly replicated the directionality and significance of associations for a large proportion of genetic loci identified until the year 2011 [12]. Therefore, despite the minor effects on risk of MS, the consistency of these results

Table 1
Overview of GWAS in multiple sclerosis and their outcomes

Study	Cases	Controls	Highlighted identified genes (non-HLA)	Novel mechanisms/insights on pathogenesis
IMSGC study, 2007 [9]	931	1862[a]	IL2RA, IL7RA	T-cell development and dysfunction of regulatory T-cells
WTCCC1 study, 2007 [58]	975	1466	USP52, SP2, PIK3R2, RAB3A	Genetic architecture in MS is shared with other autoimmune disorders
Comabella et al. [59]	242	242	Signal within intergenic locus on chromosome 13	GWA hit in linkage with functional miRNA genes
Aulchenko et al. [60]	45	195	KIF1B	Axonal loss
Baranzini et al. [61]	978	883	GPC5	Genetic diversity in genes conferring susceptibility and modifying phenotype
De Jager et al. [62]	2624 Meta-analysis (860 novel)	7220 Meta-analysis (1720 novel)	CD6, IRF8, TNFRSF1A	Interferon I signaling
ANZ gene study, 2009 [63]	1618	3413	12q13-14 region, CD40	Role of CD40 mediated regulation of humoral and cellular immunity
Sanna et al. [64]	882	872	CBLB	Defective CBLB-mediated inhibition of adaptive immune response
Nischwitz et al. [65]	590	825	No novel GWAS level significance hits	NA
Jakkula et al. [66]	68	136	STAT3	Dysregulation in Jak-STAT pathway and Th17 cell differentiation
WTCCC2 study, 2011 [11]	9772	17,376	29 Novel susceptibility loci	T-helper-cell differentiation, cell mediated immunity
Matesanz et al. [67]	296	801	No novel GWAS hits in the novel dataset, PTGER4 identified after meta-analysis with other datasets	Prostaglandin mediated inflammatory responses
Martinelli-Boneschi et al. [68]	197	234	New locus in human endogenous retroviral element	Regulation of genes involved in neurodegeneration

IMSGC International Multiple Sclerosis Genetics Consortium, *WTCCC* Wellcome Trust Case Control Consortium, *NA* not applicable
[a]Unaffected parents in trios

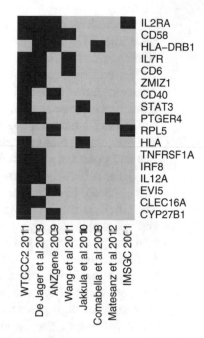

Fig. 1 Genes reaching highest concordance across GWAS tracked NHGRI catalog of GWAS studies (data extracted from: https://www.genome.gov/26525384)

clearly supports the role of the identified genetic loci in determining the heritable component of MS. It is still not clear whether such results signify that MS is a mixture of a variety of distinct neuroimmune disorders presenting with a similar phenotype, or whether it is a single condition that results from simplistic summation of multiple genetic and environmental risk factors, or whether both these hypothesis take part in disease pathogenesis. In this regard, GWAS are limited in allowing identification of genomic regions associated with MS, whereas they do not offer the possibility to distinguish between genetic variants that are causal or only genetically linked with other functionally relevant variants. Emerging technologies, including whole exome and whole genome sequencing are now widely available and open the possibility of determination of almost complete genetic constitution of an individual, and are offering promise to provide further resolution of this problem.

3 Whole-Exome Sequencing in Familiar Multiple Sclerosis

Implementation of whole-exome sequencing (WES) has successfully led to identification of genes and molecular mechanisms for several rare Mendelian disorders. A rare subset of monogenic forms has been identified in complex disorders such as Parkinson's or Alzheimer's disease. Similarly, MS may rarely run in families with several number of relatives affected which implies possibility that rare variants with high penetrance are involved in the pathogenesis of a subset of MS cases.

There have been two attempts to use WES in terms of the identification of rare variants with high impact reported so far. Ramagopalan et al. analyzed portends from 43 families with at least 4 affected members and identified rare variants in CYP27B1 gene to be associated with MS [13]. It was estimated that identified variants conferred increased risk (odds ratio = 4.7) to the disease. Furthermore, as CYP27B1 encodes the vitamin D-activating 1-alpha hydroxylase enzyme, these results support the role of vitamin D in MS pathogenesis and potential gene-environment interactions.

In another study a single MS family with 15 affected members was analyzed [14]. A rare variant of a modest effect on MS risk was identified in the TYK2 gene. The gene encodes a protein kinase that phosphorylates proteins in the JAK-STAT3 immune pathway and was predicted to interact with several genes associated with MS in GWA studies.

The two currently available studies suggest the potential of next generation sequencing in identifying genetic variants with moderate or high penetrance. Further analysis of familial and sporadic MS might significantly contribute to the understanding of the genetic contribution and mechanisms of disease.

4   Transcriptome Studies in Multiple Sclerosis

Gene expression is the most fundamental level at which an individual's genotype gives rise to the phenotype, i.e., an observable trait. With the development of high-throughput analytic methods, such as RNA microarrays and RNAseq, we are now able to study the transcriptome—a complete set of RNA transcripts produced by the genome under specific circumstances in a specific cell or tissue. The comparison of transcriptomes allows the identification of genes that are differentially expressed in distinct cell populations and consequently helps in elucidating disease mechanisms.

Given that gene expression is highly tissue specific [15], it is important to perform transcriptome studies on tissues affected by the disease being investigated. This is especially true for diseases with localized manifestations, such as MS. Although many MS transcriptome studies were performed on blood-derived samples [16], the focus of this review is on those performed on the brain, using high-throughput methods which are compatible with our hypothesis-free integratomic approach. Traditionally, MS has been considered a white matter disease on which the majority of MS brain profiling studies have been concentrated. Based on the histological analysis of demyelization, MS white matter can be divided into either normal appearing white matter (NAWM) or white matter lesions (WML). The latter are further classified as either acute (aWML), chronic active (caWML) or chronic silent (csWML), based predominantly on their infiltration with different immune

cells [17, 18]. Besides lesions in the white matter, cortical demyelination is a prominent feature of postmortem MS brains as well
[19, 20]. A general division of transcriptome studies based on tissue type analyzed can thus be made: studies analyzing WML, studies analyzing NAWM and studies analyzing gray matter. Identified
transcriptome studies are listed in Table 2.

With the aim of elucidating the mechanisms of white matter
lesion formation, the hallmark of MS, the earliest transcriptome
studies compared different lesion types with either normal appearing white matter of MS patients (NAWMms), white matter of controls without neurological disease (NAWMc) or different lesion
types amongst themselves. Different biological pathways are predominant in each cell type, thus a monotypic cell population as a
source for microarray experiments would be most desirable.
However, besides cells normally composing the white matter (oligodendrocytes, astrocytes, microglia, endothelial cells, subcortical
neurons), various lesion types are infiltrated with a different amount
and type of immune cells (T-cells, B-cells, peripheral macrophages).
The resulting expression profiles represent a complex and variable
mixture of different cell types—an overexpressed gene might be
detected due to upregulation in the resident cells or due to differences in cellularity. This warrants careful interpretation of the
results and the use of other techniques (immunohistochemistry, in
situ hybridization) to localize detected changes. Additionally, since
the identified studies are widely heterogeneous regarding lesion
types used, this contributes to the relatively poor overlap of their
results and makes them difficult to compare.

In their seminal studies Whitney and colleagues [21, 22] proposed a role of leukotrienes in the WML formation. They found a
member of the arachidonic acid (AA) cascade (LTA4 hydrolase or
arachidonate 5-lipoxygenase (5-LO)) to be overexpressed in both
of their studies. Using immunohistochemistry they localized 5-LO
predominantly to macrophages infiltrating aWML. However, the
aWML staining patterns were not specific to MS as they were
equally present in brain tissue samples from patients with cerebral
infarction, meningitis, cerebral vasculitis and carbon monoxide-
induced myelin degeneration. Although additional support for the
involvement of AA cascade is provided by overexpression of
Prostaglandin D synthase (PTGDS) in WML reported by Chabas
et al. [23], its importance remains to be proven. Besides PTGDS,
Chabas and colleagues reported alpha B-crystallin (CRYAB) as the
most abundant transcripts unique to WML. The focus of their
study, overexpression of osteopontin (OPN) however, was later
contested [24] and was not replicated by larger studies [25, 26].

Three larger studies using NAWMc for control purposes are
the most prominent in regard to WML transcriptome [25–27].
However, while Lock [25] focused on two poles of MS pathology—aWML with inflammation versus csWML, Tajouri [27]

Table 2
List of reviewed microarray based transcriptome studies performed on postmortem human brain tissue of MS patients

Study	Sample	Array size	Compared sections	Main findings
Whitney et al. [21]	1 MS (PP)	1400/5000	aWML vs. NAWMms	Inflammation related mechanisms, including LTA4 hydrolase
Whitney et al. [22]	2 MS (PP, RR), 3 Ctl (Pooled)	2798	aWML, caWML vs. NAWMc	Biosynthesis of pro-inflammatory Leukotrienes (5-LO)
Chabas et al. (EST seq study) [23]	3 MS(NA), 1 control library	Non normalized cDNA libraries	aWML vs. NAWMc	Prostaglandin D synthase, Osteopontin (confirmed with EAE) and αβ-crystallin
Lock et al. [25]	4 MS (SP), 2 Ctl	7000	aWML, caWML, csWML vs. NAWMc	Inflammatory cytokines (IL-6 and -17), MHCII, complement genes. Fcγ-receptor in inactive lesions, G-CSF in active lesions
Tajouri et al. [27]	5 MS (SP), Ctl (No. unknown)	5000	aWML, caWML vs. NAWMc	Half DEG common in all lesion types. Included identification of genes involved in response to oxidative damage
Mycko et al. [28]; Mycko et al. [29]	4 MS (SP)	588	caWML vs. csWML	Comparing margin and center of acute and chronic WML
Lindberg et al. [26]	6 MS (SP), 12 Ctl	12,000	aWML, NAWMms vs. NAWMc	Cellular immune response in NAWM, humoral immune response in lesions MS is a generalized disease
Graumann et al. [32]; Zeis et al. [33]	10 MS (SP,PP),7 Ctl	3528	NAWMms vs. NAWMc	DEG involved in Ischemic preconditioning and endogenous neuroprotection. Anti-inflammatory role of oligodendrocytes
Dutta et al. [35]; Dutta et al. [36]	6 MS (SP, PP), 6 Ctl	33,000	NAGMms vs. NAGMc	Mitochondrial dysfunction and activation of CNTF signaling pathway in neurons
Torkildsen et al. [39]	11MS (SP, PR) 12 Ctl	27,868	GML, NAGMms; vs. NAGMc	Upregulation of Ig-related genes in cortical sections
Zeis [37]	13 MS (PP,SP,PR), 8 Ctl	3528	NAGM vs. NAGMc	Reduced transcription of astrocyte specific genes involved in the ANLS and the GGC

PP primary progressive, SP secondary progressive, PR progressive relapsing, aWML/caWML/csWML acute/chronic active/chronic silent white matter lesion, NAWMms normal appearing white matter from MS patients/healthy controls, NAWMms/c normal appearing cortical gray matter from MS patients/healthy controls, GML gray matter lesion, ANLS astrocyte–neuron lactate shuttle, GGC glutamate–glutamine cycle compared aWML to caWML and Lindberg [26] focused on aWML in comparison to NAWMms. As expected, each of them found DEGs specific to particular lesion type. Tajouri emphasized that 50% of DEGs were differentially regulated in both lesion types of which only two genes (ENO2 and DPM1) were regulated in opposing directions. Similarly, Lindberg reported that 70% of sequences significantly regulated in either aWML or NAWMms showed transcriptional changes into the same direction in the respective other tissue compartment. This led both to suggest that quantitative, rather than qualitative differences in gene expression may define lesion development and evolution. According to Lindberg, lesions distinguished from NAWMms by a higher expression of genes related to immunoglobulin synthesis and neuroglial differentiation, while cellular immune response elements were equally dysregulated in both tissue compartments. Amongst other genes, Lock and colleagues identified Fc receptor common γ chain (FcγRI) and the granulocyte colony-stimulating factor (G-CSF) as uniquely differentially expressed in chronic and acute WML. Additionally, these studies identified many DEGs unspecific to lesion type. Comparing WML to NAWMc, Lock's principal finding was increased transcription of inflammatory cytokines (IL-6 and -17) and other immune-related molecules, such as histocompatibility complex (MHC) class II and complement genes. On the other hand, genes involved in the immune response represented only 21% of DEG in aWML samples analyzed by Lindberg, whereas genes operative in neural homeostasis formed the largest category (37%). Also of note is the overexpression of genes involved in response to oxidative damage (TF, SOD1, GPX1, and GSTP1) identified by Tajuri et al.

As opposed to using NAWMc for reference, direct comparison of caWML and csWML was performed in two studies [28, 29]. They demonstrated the existence of a significant difference in the transcriptional profiles of these two lesion types. Notably, an increased level of expression of adenosine A1 receptor (ADORA1) was detected in the marginal zone of the chronic active plaques. Studies on experimental autoimmune encephalitis (EAE) [30] animals depleted of the ADORA1 gene showed an increased severity of the disease course [31].

In an attempt to discover processes leading to or battling to prevent WML formation, several studies were performed comparing normal appearing white matter of MS patients (NAWMms) to NAWMc [26, 32, 33]. The main finding of the Graumann/Zeis collaboration [32, 33] was the upregulation of genes involved in the maintenance of cellular homeostasis and in neural protective mechanisms known to be induced upon long-term ischemic preconditioning and oxidative stress. Factor HIF-1alpha and associated PI3K/Akt signaling pathways, as well as their target genes, such as VEGF, were shown to be upregulated. They suggested that in MS, the brain is mounting a global defense against oxidative stress, even in areas remote from active inflammatory and demyelinating lesions, proposing a balance between oxidative stress and neural protective mechanisms. Immunohistochemistry in addition to arrays was used to show that the anti-inflammatory STAT6 signaling pathway is expressed mainly by oligodendrocytes, whereas the proinflammatory transcription factor STAT4 is expressed by microglia. This suggests that oligodendrocytes might provide anti-inflammatory environment and influence the progression of the disease. In Lindberg's study [26] the immune-related genes represented the predominant category (40%) of DEGs in NAWMms; almost double as in the aWML. Because NAWMms is defined as white matter without any pathological signs like gliosis, demyelination or infiltration, its sampling can depend upon the available methodology [34]. Two examples suggesting that NAWMms is not uniform come from Graumann's study. A striking feature was the downregulation of myelin basic protein (MBP) in many MS cases. However, in two cases, strong upregulation was detected. A feature consistent with remyelinating activity was observed (e.g., shadow plaques) in both of these cases. Another example from the same study was a MS patient that showed an expression pattern of a healthy control. This was in line with the neuropathological observation which only identified lesions in his medulla, brainstem, and spinal cord, without detecting any cortical lesions. These suggest that transcriptome abnormalities of NAWMms are anatomically or temporally related to WML which could contribute to poor reproducibility of such studies.

To identify neuronal gene changes that may contribute to axonal degeneration in chronic MS patients, several studies on their normal appearing gray matter (NAGMms) were performed. Two studies [35, 36] using the same tissue samples identified 555 DEGs. In their first publication they focused on 26 nuclear-encoded mitochondrial electron transport chain genes which were significantly underexpressed in MS samples. Reduced mitochondrial function in upper motor neurons was confirmed with functional studies which led them to suggest that a mismatch between energy demand and reduced supply of ATP causes degeneration of chronically demyelinated axons in MS patients. Using the same array dataset in their subsequent publication, they focused on 9 overexpressed genes related to ciliary neurotrophic factor (CNTF). They hypothesized that CNTF-mediated neuroprotective signaling pathway is upregulated in response to chronic insults or stress during the pathogenesis of MS. A decrease in mitochondrial function suggested by Dutta might be related to a recent transcriptome study [37]. Comparing NAGM of MS patients with the one from controls, they identified reduced transcription of astrocyte specific genes involved in the astrocyte-neuron lactate shuttle (ANLS) and the glutamate–glutamine cycle (GGC) concurrently with

Toll-like/IL-1b signaling expression signature. With additional in vitro studies and studies on mice they demonstrated that immune signaling of immune and/or central nervous system origin drives alterations in astrocytic ANLS and GGC gene regulation in the NAGM of MS patients. Since the ANLS serves to supply energetic metabolites (lactate) to neurons [38], it is possible that the down-regulation of ANLS in astrocytes is related to diminished mitochondrial function.

Another study including samples from gray matter lesions (GML) [39] found 550 DEGs. Half of IgG-related genes represented on the array were upregulated. This was probably due to presence of plasma-cell-infiltrated meningeal tissue present in the analyzed gray matter sections. No differentially expressed genes were found between normal appearing gray matter (NAGM) and gray matter lesions (GML) from MS patients. They indicated that the Ig-producing B-cells found in the cerebrospinal fluid (CSF) of MS patients could have meningeal origin.

Reviewed transcriptome studies identified many genes and associated pathways with potential roles in pathogenesis of MS, and support the concept of MS pathogenesis being a generalized process that involves the entire CNS. Besides their heterogeneity in tissue types compared, different factors such as localization of sample in the brain, stage of the lesion, amount and type of infiltration with immune cells, degeneration–regeneration ratio of the lesion, and factors pertaining to isolation procedure like the postmortem interval can influence their results. One must also consider that postmortem collecting of tissue samples meant the majority of patients were in terminal stages of secondary or primary progressive form of MS. This precludes the identification of early, potentially reversible changes leading to MS. With the development of new genetic technologies, such as single cell RNAseq [40], a more precise tissue sampling, and with it more consistent results will be achievable. Still, in order to identify pathways triggering the events that lead to MS manifestation, a precise timing of sample collection with brain biopsy would be needed to capture the events unfolding during disease onset.

5 Epigenetics in Multiple Sclerosis

Epigenetic characteristics can be defined as DNA modifications that affect the activity of genes without changing the DNA sequence. It is a way in which environmental factors may interact with genetic make-up of an individual on the regulatory level. With the development of high-throughput whole genome technologies in the last two decades, including genomic, transcriptomic and epigenomic profiling, we are now able to not only inspect epigenetic alterations in different disorders, but also to integrate interactions of various "omic" levels as well.

Three currently known epigenetic regulation mechanisms exert its effects separately, but at the same time, they are highly interrelated: (1) CpG islands methylation refers to the addition of a methyl group to the 5-position of cytosine; (2) Histone modification represents a posttranslational way of DNA regulation, where the amino-terminal tails of histones and their density can be modified; and (3) RNA-based posttranscriptional level by microRNAs (miRNA), where miRNA bind to the 3′ UTR of target mRNA, leading to mRNA cleavage or translation inhibition. The three mechanisms are directly related—DNA methylation and histone deacetylation influence miRNA expression and miRNA can regulate DNA methylation as well.

The epigenetic contribution to the pathogenesis of multiple sclerosis (MS) is beginning to be acknowledged in the last two decades—several mechanisms have already been identified in both animal models of experimental autoimmune encephalomyelitis and in humans with MS. Important piece of evidence for the contribution of epigenetics to complex diseases represent studies conducted on monozygotic twins—they share genotypes and early environment, yet they differ phenotypically by distinct susceptibility for multiple sclerosis [4, 41]. Another contributing fact was described in 2004, when it was shown that mothers significantly more often transmit multiple sclerosis to their offspring then fathers [42]. Namely, epigenetic characteristics are in general known to be inherited and transmitted in sex-specific patterns. Another interesting implication comes from the evidence that environmental factors, strongly influencing MS susceptibility, such as vitamin D levels, EBV infection and smoking [43], all have the potential to generate epigenetic changes in cells [44].

Most studied epigenetic mechanisms, shown to be important in MS, came from the studies of other autoimmune disorders and they mainly influence proinflammatory response and demyelination -remyelination steps. Both blood cells and brain specific processes have been studied and some specific changes are common to both sites. Promoter hypo or hyper-methylation, which promotes or diminishes gene expression, respectively, has been linked to differential expression of for example *PAD2*, *SHP-1*, and *IL17A in* MS patients' *peripheral blood and/or brain*. *PAD2* contributes to arginine to citrulline change in myelin basic protein, believed to predispose for autoimmunity related processes and its overexpression has been shown in MS [45]. On the contrary, downregulation of *SHP-1* expression through its promoter hypermethylation diminishes its negative regulatory role in proinflammatory signaling and therefore increases leukocyte-mediated inflammation in MS [46]. More examples are given in Table 3.

The second mechanism, histone (de)acetylation has been shown to be disrupted in MS brain tissue as well [47]. Even more, it seems that the process of histone deacetylation starts in the early

Table 3
Epigenetic studies on MS

Study	Principal finding	Downstream consequence
DNA methylation		
Mastronardi et al. [69], D'Souza et al. [70]	PAD2 promoter hypomethylation	Increased expression of PAD2 leading to increased citrullination of MBP and thereby loss of myelin stability
Makar et al. [71]	Th2 cytokine locus hypomethylation	Increased expression of IL-4, IL-5, and IL-10
Akimzhanov et al. [72]	IL-17 promoter hypermethylation	Activation of downstream gene expression
Kumagai et al. [46]	SHP-1 promoter hypermethylation	Reduced SHP-1 activity, leading to increased leukocyte-mediated inflammation
Histone modifications		
	Acetylation of white matter in frontal lobes of chronic MS patients	
Li et al. [73]	Increased H3 acetylation of mature oligodendrocytes nuclei	Increased transcriptional inhibitors of differentiation
Pedre et al. [47]	Reduced histone acetylation oligodendrocytes in early MS lesions	
Mastronardi et al. [74]	PAD4 increased histone citrullination	Reduced myelin production
Tegla et al. [75]	Decreased expression of SIRT1 in blood of MS patients	Decreased chromatin silencing through lower level of histone deacetylation
Gao et al. [76]		Increased activation of T cells
Akimzhanov et al. [72]	IL-17 promoter acetylation	Initiating chromatin accessibility for transcription factors
microRNA		
Li et al. [77]	miR-223 upregulation in blood of MS patients	Differential modulation of NF-KB pathway and central role in inflammatory responses
Junker et al. [78]	miR-34a, miR-155, miR-326 upregulation in active lesions in MS patients	All three target CD47, and therefore CD47 is reduced, thereby releasing macrophages from inhibitory control and promoting myelin phagocytosis
Noorbakhsh et al. [53]	miR-155, miR-338, miR-491 upregulation in cerebral white matter in MS patients	Suppression of levels of neurosteroids
Cox et al. [79]	miR-17, miR-20a downregulation in blood of MS patients	Changed regulation of genes involved in T cell activation

stages of the disease and histones become more and more acetylated in chronic lesions, as if the process of deacetylation would be less and less efficient. SIRT1 is a HDAC class III histone deacetylase, another protein studied in MS patients' blood and brain. Its expression was shown to be significantly decreased during disease relapses. Additional function of SIRT1 is methylation of histone H3K9, again resulting in silencing of specific genes, thereby showing interrelation of two epigenetic mechanisms. More examples are given in Table 3.

With technological advances, genome-wide data are becoming available, giving us an insight into the whole genome situation at the specific time point. Genome wide DNA methylation changes in the blood of MS patients have shown important changes in methylation patterns between different blood cell subtypes, but there were no major global changes when patients were compared to controls or when different disease subtypes were compared [48]. Detailed single CpG-site methylation investigation highlighted two CpG-sites, that were hypermethylated in all three different cell types (namely CD4+ T cells, CD8+ T cells, and white blood cells) in MS patients compared to controls. The first is located near the TMEM48 transcription start site, and the second in the APC2 exone 1. In addition, there were some CpG-sites in DNHD1 gene that were differentially methylated.

Another carefully designed study analyzed whole-genome CpG-methylation characteristics in 3 monozygotic twin-pairs discordant for MS. Again, it was shown that the biggest differences in methylation status was between different cell-types and less so between monozygotic twin sibling CD4+ lymphocytes [49].

Studies of genome wide changes in the brain unraveled 220 hypomethylated and 319 hypermethylated regions in MS affected brains, but the changes were subtle [50]. Gene ontology functional classification revealed that hypomethylated DMRs (differentially methylated regions) are highly significantly overrepresented in the categories of immune response, lymphocyte-mediated immunity, leukocyte-mediated pathways and cell killing, whereas hypermethylated DMRs are overrepresented (with lower significance) in processes such as biological regulation, actin filament-based processes, and metabolic processes.

Another mechanism of epigenetic regulation is represented by micro RNA-s (miRNA). A microRNA is a small noncoding RNA (ncRNA) molecule containing about 22 nucleotides, which functions in mRNA silencing and posttranscriptional regulation of gene expression. To date, two studies examining the profile of miRNA expression in the CNS tissue of MS patients were performed by Junker et al. and Noorbaksh et al. [51, 53]. Together they provide a signature of 50 miRNAs that are upregulated and 30 miRNAs that are downregulated in MS in comparison to healthy subjects. Interestingly, there is little overlap between miRNAs that are dysregulated in different MS lesions and normal appearing white matter (NAWM), suggesting that MS pathophysiology is heterogeneous at the level of miRNA control of gene expression. Since modified miRNA expression profiles of the sampled brain tissue may be the consequence of its infiltration with different immune cells, Junker et al. performed a laser capture micro-dissection of active lesions revealing that many upregulated miRNAs are expressed by T cells, B cells, macrophages, and astrocytes. They found three microRNAs upregulated in active multiple sclerosis lesions (microRNA-34a, microRNA-155, and microRNA-326) that target the 3'-untranslated region of CD47, which functions as a "don't eat me" signal inhibiting macrophage activity. The authors proposed that the overexpression of these three miRNAs in MS brains promotes the downregulation of CD47 on brain resident cells, thereby triggering macrophage phagocytosis of the myelin. In 2011, Noorbakhsh et al. [53] compared NAWM from MS patients and controls and demonstrated differential expression of multiple micro-RNAs, including three neurosteroid synthesis enzyme-specific micro-RNAs (miR-338, miR-155, and miR-491). Confirming their findings with functional studies, they point to impaired neurosteroidogenesis in both multiple sclerosis and experimental autoimmune encephalomyelitis.

These studies show that miRNA-s are involved in the misregulated immune system in MS, however, many more studies will be needed before their role in MS will be elucidated.

With new genome technologies it is now possible to analyzes the whole-genome epigenetic status, an epigenome, instead of studying preselected genes or regions. Epigenetic marks tightly regulate transcription, therefore, combined studies of epigenomic and transcriptomic (genome-wide gene expression) signatures would be of great importance. This approach enables us to validate direct effects of epigenetic changes on gene expression.

Even more promising is the potential therapeutic intervention through modifying the epigenome. Epigenetic modifications are, as we know, reversible and dynamic characteristics and with their regulation it is possible to fine-tune therapies, namely, specific therapeutic compounds have the ability to influence DNA methylation status and hence transcriptional activity. Before this could be of clinical use we need to understand the effects of the epigenome in the MS susceptibility and progression.

6   Integrative View of Results from Omic Studies in Multiple Sclerosis

Complex and heterogeneous nature of etiologic and pathogenetic processes in MS presents a significant challenge in fully characterizing the causes and modifying factors in MS. Although various omic approaches offer a comprehensive insight in identifying molecular alterations in multiple sclerosis, they are limited by issues stemming from testing multiple hypotheses, failures to replicate the significant findings and limited ability to distinguish statistical noise from a consistent biological signal. Advancement in understanding MS thus requires comprehensive understanding of the interplay of various omic layers as they occur in actual biological systems.

Aiming to precipitate the alterations that are consistently reflected across omic levels, we previously outlined an approach that enables streamlined integration of heterogeneous information, which is based on detection of genomic regions with clustering of biological signals from various omic levels. Comparison of cross-omic convergence of hits in multiple sclerosis has identified several regions where at least two distinct types of omic hits support involvement of these regions in the pathogenesis of multiple sclerosis, and identified several novel hits that have previously been lost amidst the statistical noise.

Investigating results from studies presented in this article show that several genes in GWAS regions display differential mRNA or protein expression in brain transcriptome profiling studies (RGS1, IL7R, EXTL2, SORBS2, MERTK, DDAH1, LMAN2, DIAPH1, ARHGEF3), offering functional explanation for contained genetic variants through gene expression regulation. There is also a notable concordance of results between transcriptome studies and proteome level studies—for at least 23 genes differentially expressed genes in MS, their protein product could be found specifically in active inflammatory plaques of patients with MS.

Interestingly, cross-omic analysis also shows that a number of genes differentially expressed in MS contain sequence targets of microRNA molecules shown to be dysregulated in multiple sclerosis. As an example, PER3 gene has been distinctly identified in active MS plaques [53] and also is regulated by miR-30a microRNA that is concurrently dysregulated in active MS plaques.

Investigation of data originating from multi-omic sources defines perturbations in gene networks that may not be evident from separate analysis of a single layer. In this manner, ensemble analysis precipitates the role of Jak-STAT pathway in MS, which is supported by evidence from various omic layers. It is known that its deregulation has been consistently implicated in a variety of autoimmune disorders, due to disinhibition of regulatory cytokines in the inflammatory process. In addition to the support from omics studies, several other lines of evidence have now been collected that support the crucial role of JAK-STAT pathway in multiple sclerosis. In particular, expression of STAT3, a core player in the STAT signaling pathway, has been found increased in T-cells from patients during the relapse episodes and high STAT3 expression levels have been found to affect progression to fully developed MS syndrome [54, 55]. Further evidence comes from animal models, where abolishment of STAT3 activity in T-cells protects mice

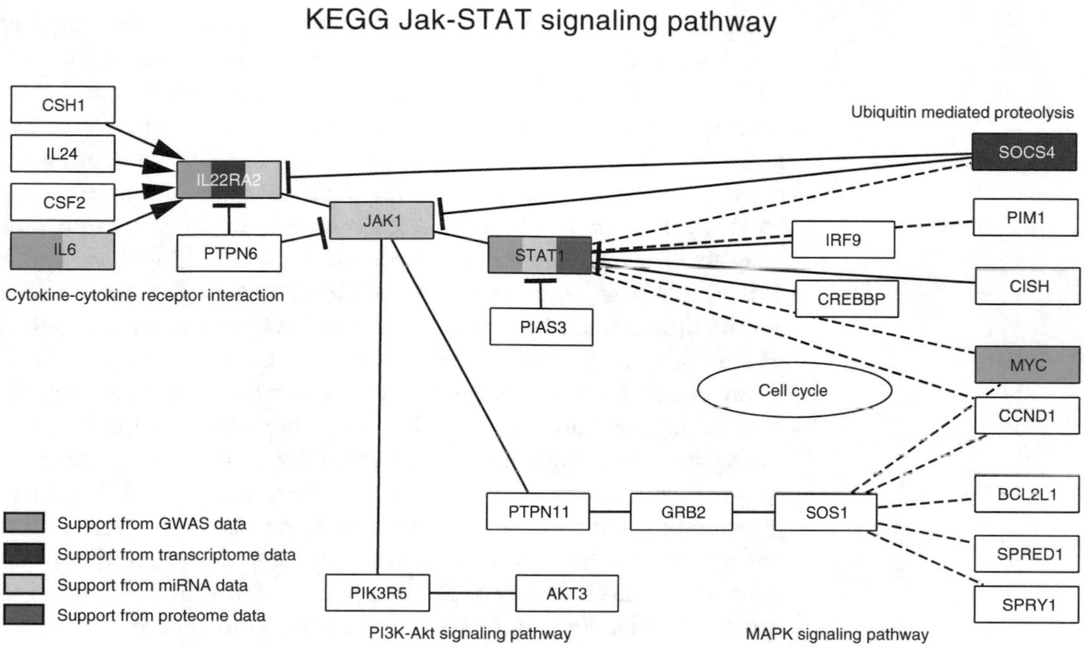

KEGG Jak-STAT signaling pathway

Fig. 2 Confluence of results from various omic levels in support of the role of Jak-STAT signaling pathway deregulation in MS. Signals from four different omic layers delineate alterations in several key nodes of the pathway, where the deregulation may not be present in the same gene, but colocalizes to the same functional network

from developing the experimental autoimmune encephalitis (EAE) [30]. Several studies have also shown therapeutic promise with agents targeting JAK-STAT pathway. Studies on animal models have shown that JAK inhibitors were able to reduce the severity of EAE in mice [56]. Furthermore, recent evidence suggests that in EAE models, JAK1/2 inhibitors were able to reduce the entry of immune cells into the central nervous system, inhibit differentiation of myeloid cells to Th1 and Th17 lineage, inhibiting STAT activation in brain and generally reduce the expression of proinflammatory cytokines [57].

This and similar examples show how the convergence of results from omic profiling studies can thus provide meaningful biological clues, not only when overlapping results obtained on the same biological level, but also when combining signals originating from a variety of biological levels (Fig. 2).

7 Conclusion

The etiology of multiple sclerosis, a relatively common chronic inflammatory neurodegenerative disease of the CNS, is still largely unknown. It is considered as a multifactorial disease, where complex interplay of genes and environment increase susceptibility for the disease and direct its subtype and progression. Genome-wide association studies and exome sequencing revealed and convincingly replicated a few genetic loci with a modest impact on MS and some more with a minor influence, thereby confirming an existing heritable component of MS. Such genome-wide approaches to study human health and disease enable us to get important insights into the changes and characteristics on a global scale, but at the same time, some genome-wide level studies give inconsistent results between studies. Epigenomic and transcriptomic studies in MS revealed important disease related changes, but studies of different research groups often failed to replicate the results, partially due to highly sensitive and tissue specific mechanisms of gene expression and epigenome characteristics and partially because these are influenced on by daily habits, diet, and stress. Using integratomic approaches we are now able to combine all these different genome-wide levels to search for the common disturbed mechanism and this approach already proved useful by identifying specific cellular signaling pathways, disturbed in MS. With further technological and knowledge development, use of systems biology and whole genome sequencing and performing larger studies, the future promises to bring answers to many open questions.

References

1. Ascherio A (2013) Environmental factors in multiple sclerosis. Expert Rev Neurother 13(12 Suppl):3–9. doi:10.1586/14737175.2013.865866

2. Marrie RA, Cohen J, Stuve O, Trojano M, Sorensen PS, Reingold S, Cutter G, Reider N (2015) A systematic review of the incidence and prevalence of comorbidity in multiple sclerosis: overview. Mult Scler 21(3):263–281. doi:10.1177/1352458514564491

3. Dyment DA, Yee IM, Ebers GC, Sadovnick AD, Canadian Collaborative Study Group (2006) Multiple sclerosis in stepsiblings: recurrence risk and ascertainment. J Neurol Neurosurg Psychiatry 77(2):258–259. doi:10.1136/jnnp.2005.063008

4. O'Gorman C, Lin R, Stankovich J, Broadley SA (2013) Modelling genetic susceptibility to multiple sclerosis with family data. Neuroepidemiology 40(1):1–12. doi:10.1159/000341902

5. Simpson S Jr, Taylor BV, van der Mei I (2015) The role of epidemiology in MS research: past successes, current challenges and future potential. Mult Scler 21(8):969–977. doi:10.1177/1352458515574896

6. Naito S, Namerow N, Mickey MR, Terasaki PI (1972) Multiple sclerosis: association with HL-A3. Tissue Antigens 2(1):1–4

7. Oksenberg JR, Baranzini SE (2010) Multiple sclerosis genetics—is the glass half full, or half empty? Nat Rev Neurol 6(8):429–437. doi:10.1038/nrneurol.2010.91

8. Sawcer S, Franklin RJ, Ban M (2014) Multiple sclerosis genetics. Lancet Neurol 13(7):700–709. doi:10.1016/S1474-4422(14)70041-9

9. International Multiple Sclerosis Genetics Consortium, Hafler DA, Compston A, Sawcer S, Lander ES, Daly MJ, De Jager PL, de Bakker PI, Gabriel SB, Mirel DB, Ivinson AJ, Pericak-Vance MA, Gregory SG, Rioux JD, McCauley JL, Haines JL, Barcellos LF, Cree B, Oksenberg JR, Hauser SL (2007) Risk alleles for multiple sclerosis identified by a genome-wide study. N Engl J Med 357(9):851–862, doi: NEJMoa073493 [pii] 10.1056/NEJMoa073493

10. Hartmann FJ, Khademi M, Aram J, Ammann S, Kockum I, Constantinescu C, Gran B, Piehl F, Olsson T, Codarri L, Becher B (2014) Multiple sclerosis-associated IL2RA polymorphism controls GM-CSF production in human

TH cells. Nat Commun 5:5056. doi:10.1038/ncomms6056

11. International Multiple Sclerosis Genetics Consortium, Wellcome Trust Case Control Consortium, Sawcer S, Hellenthal G, Pirinen M, Spencer CC, Patsopoulos NA, Moutsianas L, Dilthey A, Su Z, Freeman C, Hunt SE, Edkins S, Gray E, Booth DR, Potter SC, Goris A, Band G, Oturai AB, Strange A, Saarela J, Bellenguez C, Fontaine B, Gillman M, Hemmer B, Gwilliam R, Zipp F, Jayakumar A, Martin R, Leslie S, Hawkins S, Giannoulatou E, D'Alfonso S, Blackburn H, Martinelli Boneschi F, Liddle J, Harbo HF, Perez ML, Spurkland A, Waller MJ, Mycko MP, Ricketts M, Comabella M, Hammond N, Kockum I, McCann OT, Ban M, Whittaker P, Kemppinen A, Weston P, Hawkins C, Widaa S, Zajicek J, Dronov S, Robertson N, Bumpstead SJ, Barcellos LF, Ravindrarajah R, Abraham R, Alfredsson L, Ardlie K, Aubin C, Baker A, Baker K, Baranzini SE, Bergamaschi L, Bergamaschi R, Bernstein A, Berthele A, Boggild M, Bradfield JP, Brassat D, Broadley SA, Buck D, Butzkueven H, Capra R, Carroll WM, Cavalla P, Celius EG, Cepok S, Chiavacci R, Clerget-Darpoux F, Clysters K, Comi G, Cossburn M, Cournu-Rebeix I, Cox MB, Cozen W, Cree BA, Cross AH, Cusi D, Daly MJ, Davis E, de Bakker PI, Debouverie M, D'Hooghe MB, Dixon K, Dobosi R, Dubois B, Ellinghaus D, Elovaara I, Esposito F, Fontenille C, Foote S, Franke A, Galimberti D, Ghezzi A, Glessner J, Gomez R, Gout O, Graham C, Grant SF, Guerini FR, Hakonarson H, Hall P, Hamsten A, Hartung HP, Heard RN, Heath S, Hobart J, Hoshi M, Infante-Duarte C, Ingram G, Ingram W, Islam T, Jagodic M, Kabesch M, Kermode AG, Kilpatrick TJ, Kim C, Klopp N, Koivisto K, Larsson M, Lathrop M, Lechner-Scott JS, Leone MA, Leppa V, Liljedahl U, Bomfim IL, Lincoln RR, Link J, Liu J, Lorentzen AR, Lupoli S, Macciardi F, Mack T, Marriott M, Martinelli V, Mason D, McCauley JL, Mentch F, Mero IL, Mihalova T, Montalban X, Mottershead J, Myhr KM, Naldi P, Ollier W, Page A, Palotie A, Pelletier J, Piccio L, Pickersgill T, Piehl F, Pobywajlo S, Quach HL, Ramsay PP, Reunanen M, Reynolds R, Rioux JD, Rodegher M, Roesner S, Rubio JP, Ruckert IM, Salvetti M, Salvi E, Santaniello A, Schaefer CA, Schreiber S, Schulze C, Scott RJ, Sellebjerg F, Selmaj KW, Sexton D, Shen L, Simms-Acuna B, Skidmore S, Sleiman PM, Smestad C, Sorensen PS, Sondergaard HB, Stankovich J, Strange RC, Sulonen AM, Sundqvist E, Syvanen AC, Taddeo F, Taylor B, Blackwell JM, Tienari P, Bramon E, Tourbah A, Brown MA, Tronczynska E, Casas JP, Tubridy N, Corvin A, Vickery J, Jankowski J, Villoslada P, Markus HS, Wang K, Mathew CG, Wason J, Palmer CN, Wichmann HE, Plomin R, Willoughby E, Rautanen A, Winkelmann J, Wittig M, Trembath RC, Yaouanq J, Viswanathan AC, Zhang H, Wood NW, Zuvich R, Deloukas P, Langford C, Duncanson A, Oksenberg JR, Pericak-Vance MA, Haines JL, Olsson T, Hillert J, Ivinson AJ, De Jager PL, Peltonen L, Stewart GJ, Hafler DA, Hauser SL, McVean G, Donnelly P, Compston A (2011) Genetic risk and a primary role for cell-mediated immune mechanisms in multiple sclerosis. Nature 476(7359):214–219. doi:10.1038/nature10251

12. International Multiple Sclerosis Genetics Consortium, Beecham AH, Patsopoulos NA, Xifara DK, Davis MF, Kemppinen A, Cotsapas C, Shah TS, Spencer C, Booth D, Goris A, Oturai A, Saarela J, Fontaine B, Hemmer B, Martin C, Zipp F, D'Alfonso S, Martinelli-Boneschi F, Taylor B, Harbo HF, Kockum I, Hillert J, Olsson T, Ban M, Oksenberg JR, Hintzen R, Barcellos LF, Wellcome Trust Case Control C, International IBDGC, Agliardi C, Alfredsson L, Alizadeh M, Anderson C, Andrews R, Sondergaard HB, Baker A, Band G, Baranzini SE, Barizzone N, Barrett J, Bellenguez C, Bergamaschi L, Bernardinelli L, Berthele A, Biberacher V, Binder TM, Blackburn H, Bomfim II, Brambilla P, Broadley S, Brochet B, Brundin L, Buck D, Butzkueven H, Caillier SJ, Camu W, Carpenter W, Cavalla P, Celius EG, Coman I, Comi G, Corrado L, Cosemans L, Cournu-Rebeix I, Cree BA, Cusi D, Damotte V, Defer G, Delgado SR, Deloukas P, di Sapio A, Dilthey AT, Donnelly P, Dubois B, Duddy M, Edkins S, Elovaara I, Esposito F, Evangelou N, Fiddes B, Field J, Franke A, Freeman C, Frohlich IY, Galimberti D, Gieger C, Gourraud PA, Graetz C, Graham A, Grummel V, Guaschino C, Hadjixenofontos A, Hakonarson H, Halfpenny C, Hall G, Hall P, Hamsten A, Harley J, Harrower T, Hawkins C, Hellenthal G, Hillier C, Hobart J, Hoshi M, Hunt SE, Jagodic M, Jelcic I, Jochim A, Kendall B, Kermode A, Kilpatrick T, Koivisto K, Konidari I, Korn T, Kronsbein H, Langford C, Larsson M, Lathrop M, Lebrun-Frenay C, Lechner-Scott J, Lee MH, Leone MA, Leppa V, Liberatore G, Lie BA, Lill CM, Linden M, Link J, Luessi F, Lycke J, Macciardi F, Mannisto S, Manrique CP, Martin R, Martinelli V, Mason D, Mazibrada G, McCabe C, Mero IL, Mescheriakova J, Moutsianas L, Myhr KM, Nagels G, Nicholas R, Nilsson P, Piehl F, Pirinen M, Price SE, Quach H, Reunanen M, Robberecht W, Robertson NP, Rodegher M, Rog D, Salvetti M, Schnetz-Boutaud NC, Sellebjerg F, Selter RC, Schaefer C, Shaunak S,

Shen L, Shields S, Siffrin V, Slee M, Sorensen PS, Sorosina M, Sospedra M, Spurkland A, Strange A, Sundqvist E, Thijs V, Thorpe J, Ticca A, Tienari P, van Duijn C, Visser EM, Vucic S, Westerlind H, Wiley JS, Wilkins A, Wilson JF, Winkelmann J, Zajicek J, Zindler E, Haines JL, Pericak-Vance MA, Ivinson AJ, Stewart G, Hafler D, Hauser SL, Compston A, McVean G, De Jager P, Sawcer SJ, McCauley JL (2013) Analysis of immune-related loci identifies 48 new susceptibility variants for multiple sclerosis. Nat Genet 45(11):1353–1360. doi:10.1038/ng.2770

13. Ramagopalan SV, Dyment DA, Cader MZ, Morrison KM, Disanto G, Morahan JM, Berlanga-Taylor AJ, Handel A, De Luca GC, Sadovnick AD, Lepage P, Montpetit A, Ebers GC (2011) Rare variants in the CYP27B1 gene are associated with multiple sclerosis. Ann Neurol 70(6):881–886. doi:10.1002/ana.22678

14. Dyment DA, Cader MZ, Chao MJ, Lincoln MR, Morrison KM, Disanto G, Morahan JM, De Luca GC, Sadovnick AD, Lepage P, Montpetit A, Ebers GC, Ramagopalan SV (2012) Exome sequencing identifies a novel multiple sclerosis susceptibility variant in the TYK2 gene. Neurology 79(5):406–411. doi:10.1212/WNL.0b013e3182616fc4

15. Mele M, Ferreira PG, Reverter F, DeLuca DS, Monlong J, Sammeth M, Young TR, Goldmann JM, Pervouchine DD, Sullivan TJ, Johnson R, Segre AV, Djebali S, Niarchou A, Consortium GT, Wright FA, Lappalainen T, Calvo M, Getz G, Dermitzakis ET, Ardlie KG, Guigo R (2015) Human genomics. the human transcriptome across tissues and individuals. Science 348(6235):660–665. doi:10.1126/science.aaa0355

16. Kemppinen AK, Kaprio J, Palotie A, Saarela J (2011) Systematic review of genome-wide expression studies in multiple sclerosis. BMJ Open 1(1), e000053. doi:10.1136/bmjopen-2011-000053

17. Trapp BD, Peterson J, Ransohoff RM, Rudick R, Mork S, Bo L (1998) Axonal transection in the lesions of multiple sclerosis. N Engl J Med 338(5):278–285. doi:10.1056/NEJM199801293380502

18. van der Valk P, De Groot CJ (2000) Staging of multiple sclerosis (MS) lesions: pathology of the time frame of MS. Neuropathol Appl Neurobiol 26(1):2–10

19. Kidd D, Barkhof F, McConnell R, Algra PR, Allen IV, Revesz T (1999) Cortical lesions in multiple sclerosis. Brain 122(Pt 1):17–26

20. Kutzelnigg A, Lassmann H (2005) Cortical lesions and brain atrophy in MS. J Neurol Sci 233(1–2):55–59. doi:10.1016/j.jns.2005.03.027

21. Whitney LW, Becker KG, Tresser NJ, Caballero-Ramos CI, Munson PJ, Prabhu VV, Trent JM, McFarland HF, Biddison WE (1999) Analysis of gene expression in multiple sclerosis lesions using cDNA microarrays. Ann Neurol 46(3):425–428

22. Whitney LW, Ludwin SK, McFarland HF, Biddison WE (2001) Microarray analysis of gene expression in multiple sclerosis and EAE identifies 5-lipoxygenase as a component of inflammatory lesions. J Neuroimmunol 121(1–2):40–48

23. Chabas D, Baranzini SE, Mitchell D, Bernard CC, Rittling SR, Denhardt DT, Sobel RA, Lock C, Karpuj M, Pedotti R, Heller R, Oksenberg JR, Steinman L (2001) The influence of the proinflammatory cytokine, osteopontin, on autoimmune demyelinating disease. Science 294(5547):1731–1735. doi:10.1126/science.1062960

24. Blom T, Franzen A, Heinegard D, Holmdahl R (2003) Comment on "The influence of the proinflammatory cytokine, osteopontin, on autoimmune demyelinating disease". Science 299(5614):1845. doi:10.1126/science.1078985, author reply 1845

25. Lock C, Hermans G, Pedotti R, Brendolan A, Schadt E, Garren H, Langer-Gould A, Strober S, Cannella B, Allard J, Klonowski P, Austin A, Lad N, Kaminski N, Galli SJ, Oksenberg JR, Raine CS, Heller R, Steinman L (2002) Gene-microarray analysis of multiple sclerosis lesions yields new targets validated in autoimmune encephalomyelitis. Nat Med 8(5):500–508. doi:10.1038/nm0502-500

26. Lindberg RL, De Groot CJ, Certa U, Ravid R, Hoffmann F, Kappos L, Leppert D (2004) Multiple sclerosis as a generalized CNS disease—comparative microarray analysis of normal appearing white matter and lesions in secondary progressive MS. J Neuroimmunol 152(1–2):154–167. doi:10.1016/j.jneuroim.2004.03.011

27. Tajouri L, Mellick AS, Ashton KJ, Tannenberg AEG, Nagra RM, Tourtellotte WW, Griffiths LR (2003) Quantitative and qualitative changes in gene expression patterns characterize the activity of plaques in multiple sclerosis. Mol Brain Res 119(2):170–183. doi:10.1016/j.molbrainres.2003.09.008

28. Mycko MP, Papoian R, Boschert U, Raine CS, Selmaj KW (2003) cDNA microarray analysis in multiple sclerosis lesions: detection of genes associated with disease activity. Brain 126(Pt 5):1048–1057

29. Mycko MP, Papoian R, Boschert U, Raine CS, Selmaj KW (2004) Microarray gene

expression profiling of chronic active and inactive lesions in multiple sclerosis. Clin Neurol Neurosurg 106(3):223–229. doi:10.1016/j.clineuro.2004.02.019

30. Liu X, Lee YS, Yu CR, Egwuagu CE (2008) Loss of STAT3 in CD4+ T cells prevents development of experimental autoimmune diseases. J Immunol 180(9):6070–6076

31. Tsutsui S, Schnermann J, Noorbakhsh F, Henry S, Yong VW, Winston BW, Warren K, Power C (2004) A1 adenosine receptor upregulation and activation attenuates neuroinflammation and demyelination in a model of multiple sclerosis. J Neurosci 24(6):1521–1529. doi:10.1523/JNEUROSCI.4271-03.2004

32. Graumann U, Reynolds R, Steck AJ, Schaeren-Wiemers N (2003) Molecular changes in normal appearing white matter in multiple sclerosis are characteristic of neuroprotective mechanisms against hypoxic insult. Brain Pathol 13(4):554–573

33. Zeis T, Graumann U, Reynolds R, Schaeren-Wiemers N (2008) Normal-appearing white matter in multiple sclerosis is in a subtle balance between inflammation and neuroprotection. Brain 131(Pt 1):288–303. doi:10.1093/brain/awm291

34. Allen IV, McKeown SR (1979) A histological, histochemical and biochemical study of the macroscopically normal white matter in multiple sclerosis. J Neurol Sci 41(1):81–91

35. Dutta R, McDonough J, Yin X, Peterson J, Chang A, Torres T, Gudz T, Macklin WB, Lewis DA, Fox RJ, Rudick R, Mirnics K, Trapp BD (2006) Mitochondrial dysfunction as a cause of axonal degeneration in multiple sclerosis patients. Ann Neurol 59(3):478–489. doi:10.1002/ana.20736

36. Dutta R, McDonough J, Chang A, Swamy L, Siu A, Kidd GJ, Rudick R, Mirnics K, Trapp BD (2007) Activation of the ciliary neurotrophic factor (CNTF) signalling pathway in cortical neurons of multiple sclerosis patients. Brain 130(Pt 10):2566–2576. doi:10.1093/brain/awm206

37. Zeis T, Allaman I, Gentner M, Schroder K, Tschopp J, Magistretti PJ, Schaeren-Wiemers N (2015) Metabolic gene expression changes in astrocytes in multiple sclerosis cerebral cortex are indicative of immune-mediated signaling. Brain Behav Immun. doi: 10.1016/j.bbi.2015.04.013

38. Pellerin L, Magistretti PJ (2012) Sweet sixteen for ANLS. J Cereb Blood Flow Metab 32(7):1152–1166. doi:10.1038/jcbfm.2011.149

39. Torkildsen O, Stansberg C, Angelskar SM, Kooi EJ, Geurts JJ, van der Valk P, Myhr KM, Steen VM, Bo L (2010) Upregulation of immunoglobulin-related genes in cortical sections from multiple sclerosis patients. Brain Pathol 20(4):720–729. doi:10.1111/j.1750-3639.2009.00343.x

40. Chepelev I, Wei G, Tang Q, Zhao K (2009) Detection of single nucleotide variations in expressed exons of the human genome using RNA-Seq. Nucleic Acids Res 37(16), e106. doi:10.1093/nar/gkp507

41. Kucukali CI, Kurtuncu M, Coban A, Cebi M, Tuzun E (2015) Epigenetics of multiple sclerosis: an updated review. Neuromolecular Med 17(2):83–96. doi:10.1007/s12017-014-8298-6

42. Ebers GC, Sadovnick AD, Dyment DA, Yee IM, Willer CJ, Risch N (2004) Parent-of-origin effect in multiple sclerosis: observations in half-siblings. Lancet 363(9423):1773–1774. doi:10.1016/S0140-6736(04)16304-6

43. Ramagopalan SV, Dobson R, Meier UC, Giovannoni G (2010) Multiple sclerosis: risk factors, prodromes, and potential causal pathways. Lancet Neurol 9(7):727–739. doi:10.1016/S1474-4422(10)70094-6

44. Niller HH, Tarnai Z, Decsi G, Zsedenyi A, Banati F, Minarovits J (2014) Role of epigenetics in EBV regulation and pathogenesis. Future Microbiol 9(6):747–756. doi:10.2217/fmb.14.41

45. Calabrese R, Zampieri M, Mechelli R, Annibali V, Guastafierro T, Ciccarone F, Coarelli G, Umeton R, Salvetti M, Caiafa P (2012) Methylation-dependent PAD2 upregulation in multiple sclerosis peripheral blood. Mult Scler 18(3):299–304. doi:10.1177/1352458511421055

46. Kumagai C, Kalman B, Middleton FA, Vyshkina T, Massa PT (2012) Increased promoter methylation of the immune regulatory gene SHP-1 in leukocytes of multiple sclerosis subjects. J Neuroimmunol 246(1–2):51–57. doi:10.1016/j.jneuroim.2012.03.003

47. Pedre X, Mastronardi F, Bruck W, Lopez-Rodas G, Kuhlmann T, Casaccia P (2011) Changed histone acetylation patterns in normal-appearing white matter and early multiple sclerosis lesions. J Neurosci 31(9):3435–3445. doi:10.1523/JNEUROSCI.4507-10.2011

48. Bos SD, Page CM, Andreassen BK, Elboudwarej E, Gustavsen MW, Briggs F, Quach H, Leikfoss IS, Bjolgerud A, Berge T, Harbo HF, Barcellos LF (2015) Genome-wide DNA methylation profiles indicate CD8+ T cell hypermethylation in multiple sclerosis. PLoS One 10(3):e0117403. doi:10.1371/journal.pone.0117403

49. Baranzini SE, Mudge J, van Velkinburgh JC, Khankhanian P, Khrebtukova I, Miller NA, Zhang L, Farmer AD, Bell CJ, Kim RW, May

GD, Woodward JE, Caillier SJ, McElroy JP, Gomez R, Pando MJ, Clendenen LE, Ganusova EE, Schilkey FD, Ramaraj T, Khan OA, Huntley JJ, Luo S, Kwok PY, Wu TD, Schroth GP, Oksenberg JR, Hauser SL, Kingsmore SF (2010) Genome, epigenome and RNA sequences of monozygotic twins discordant for multiple sclerosis. Nature 464(7293):1351–1356. doi:10.1038/nature08990

50. Huynh JL, Garg P, Thin TH, Yoo S, Dutta R, Trapp BD, Haroutunian V, Zhu J, Donovan MJ, Sharp AJ, Casaccia P (2014) Epigenome-wide differences in pathology-free regions of multiple sclerosis-affected brains. Nat Neurosci 17(1):121–130. doi:10.1038/nn.3588

51. Junker JP, Ziegler F, Rief M (2009) Ligand-dependent equilibrium fluctuations of single calmodulin molecules. Science 323(5914):633–637. doi:10.1126/science.1166191

52. Noorbakhsh F, Ellestad KK, Maingat F, Warren KG, Han MH, Steinman L, Baker GB, Power C (2011) Impaired neurosteroid synthesis in multiple sclerosis. Brain 134(Pt 9):2703–2721. doi:10.1093/brain/awr200

53. Han MH, Hwang SI, Roy DB, Lundgren DH, Price JV, Ousman SS, et al (2008) Proteomic analysis of active multiple sclerosis lesions reveals therapeutic targets. Nature. 451:1076.

54. Frisullo G, Angelucci F, Caggiula M, Nociti V, Iorio R, Patanella AK, Sancricca C, Mirabella M, Tonali PA, Batocchi AP (2006) pSTAT1, pSTAT3, and T-bet expression in peripheral blood mononuclear cells from relapsing-remitting multiple sclerosis patients correlates with disease activity. J Neurosci Res 84(5):1027–1036. doi:10.1002/jnr.20995

55. Frisullo G, Nociti V, Iorio R, Patanella AK, Marti A, Mirabella M, Tonali PA, Batocchi AP (2008) The persistency of high levels of pSTAT3 expression in circulating CD4+ T cells from CIS patients favors the early conversion to clinically defined multiple sclerosis. J Neuroimmunol 205(1–2):126–134. doi:10.1016/j.jneuroim.2008.09.003

56. Bright JJ, Du C, Sriram S (1999) Tyrphostin B42 inhibits IL-12-induced tyrosine phosphorylation and activation of Janus kinase-2 and prevents experimental allergic encephalomyelitis. J Immunol 162(10):6255–6262

57. Liu Y, Holdbrooks AT, De Sarno P, Rowse AL, Yanagisawa LL, McFarland BC, Harrington LE, Raman C, Sabbaj S, Benveniste EN, Qin H (2014) Therapeutic efficacy of suppressing the Jak/STAT pathway in multiple models of experimental autoimmune encephalomyelitis. J Immunol 192(1):59–72. doi:10.4049/jimmunol.1301513

58. Wellcome Trust Case Control Consortium, Australo-Anglo-American Spondylitis Consortium Burton PR, Clayton DG, Cardon LR, Craddock N, Deloukas P, Duncanson A, Kwiatkowski DP, McCarthy MI, Ouwehand WH, Samani NJ, Todd JA, Donnelly P, Barrett JC, Davison D, Easton D, Evans DM, Leung HT, Marchini JL, Morris AP, Spencer CC, Tobin MD, Attwood AP, Boorman JP, Cant B, Everson U, Hussey JM, Jolley JD, Knight AS, Koch K, Meech E, Nutland S, Prowse CV, Stevens HE, Taylor NC, Walters GR, Walker NM, Watkins NA, Winzer T, Jones RW, McArdle WL, Ring SM, Strachan DP, Pembrey M, Breen G, St Clair D, Caesar S, Gordon-Smith K, Jones L, Fraser C, Green EK, Grozeva D, Hamshere ML, Holmans PA, Jones IR, Kirov G, Moskivina V, Nikolov I, O'Donovan MC, Owen MJ, Collier DA, Elkin A, Farmer A, Williamson R, McGuffin P, Young AH, Ferrier IN, Ball SG, Balmforth AJ, Barrett JH, Bishop TD, Iles MM, Maqbool A, Yuldasheva N, Hall AS, Braund PS, Dixon RJ, Mangino M, Stevens S, Thompson JR, Bredin F, Tremelling M, Parkes M, Drummond H, Lees CW, Nimmo ER, Satsangi J, Fisher SA, Forbes A, Lewis CM, Onnie CM, Prescott NJ, Sanderson J, Matthew CG, Barbour J, Mohiuddin MK, Todhunter CE, Mansfield JC, Ahmad T, Cummings FR, Jewell DP, Webster J, Brown MJ, Lathrop MG, Connell J, Dominiczak A, Marcano CA, Burke B, Dobson R, Gungadoo J, Lee KL, Munroe PB, Newhouse SJ, Onipinla A, Wallace C, Xue M, Caulfield M, Farrall M, Barton A, Biologics in RAG, Genomics Study Syndicate Steering C, Bruce IN, Donovan H, Eyre S, Gilbert PD, Hilder SL, Hinks AM, John SL, Potter C, Silman AJ, Symmons DP, Thomson W, Worthington J, Dunger DB, Widmer B, Frayling TM, Freathy RM, Lango H, Perry JR, Shields BM, Weedon MN, Hattersley AT, Hitman GA, Walker M, Elliott KS, Groves CJ, Lindgren CM, Rayner NW, Timpson NJ, Zeggini E, Newport M, Sirugo G, Lyons E, Vannberg F, Hill AV, Bradbury LA, Farrar C, Pointon JJ, Wordsworth P, Brown MA, Franklyn JA, Heward JM, Simmonds MJ, Gough SC, Seal S, Breast Cancer Susceptibility C, Stratton MR, Rahman N, Ban M, Goris A, Sawcer SJ, Compston A, Conway D, Jallow M, Newport M, Sirugo G, Rockett KA, Bumpstead SJ, Chaney A, Downes K, Ghori MJ, Gwilliam R, Hunt SE, Inouye M, Keniry A, King E, McGinnis R, Potter S, Ravindrarajah R, Whittaker P, Widden C, Withers D, Cardin NJ, Davison D, Ferreira T, Pereira-Gale J, Hallgrimsdo'ttir IB, Howie BN, Su Z, Teo YY, Vukcevic D, Bentley D, Brown MA, Compston A, Farrall M, Hall AS, Hattersley AT, Hill AV, Parkes M, Pembrey M, Stratton MR, Mitchell SL, Newby PR, Brand OJ, Carr-Smith J, Pearce SH, McGinnis R, Keniry A, Deloukas P, Reveille JD, Zhou

X, Sims AM, Dowling A, Taylor J, Doan T, Davis JC, Savage L, Ward MM, Learch TL, Weisman MH, Brown M (2007) Association scan of 14,500 nonsynonymous SNPs in four diseases identifies autoimmunity variants. Nat Genet 39(11):1329–1337. doi: 10.1038/ng.2007.17

59. Comabella M, Craig DW, Camina-Tato M, Morcillo C, Lopez C, Navarro A, Rio J, Biomarker MSSG, Montalban X, Martin R (2008) Identification of a novel risk locus for multiple sclerosis at 13q31.3 by a pooled genome-wide scan of 500,000 single nucleotide polymorphisms. PLoS One 3(10):e3490, doi: 10.1371/journal.pone.0003490

60. Aulchenko YS, Hoppenbrouwers IA, Ramagopalan SV, Broer L, Jafari N, Hillert J, Link J, Lundstrom W, Greiner E, Dessa Sadovnick A, Goossens D, Van Broeckhoven C, Del-Favero J, Ebers GC, Oostra BA, van Duijn CM, Hintzen RQ (2008) Genetic variation in the KIF1B locus influences susceptibility to multiple sclerosis. Nat Genet 40(12):1402–1403. doi:10.1038/ng.251

61. Baranzini SE, Wang J, Gibson RA, Galwey N, Naegelin Y, Barkhof F, Radue EW, Lindberg RL, Uitdehaag BM, Johnson MR, Angelakopoulou A, Hall L, Richardson JC, Prinjha RK, Gass A, Geurts JJ, Kragt J, Sombekke M, Vrenken H, Qualley P, Lincoln RR, Gomez R, Caillier SJ, George MF, Mousavi H, Guerrero R, Okuda DT, Cree BA, Green AJ, Waubant E, Goodin DS, Pelletier D, Matthews PM, Hauser SL, Kappos L, Polman CH, Oksenberg JR (2009) Genome-wide association analysis of susceptibility and clinical phenotype in multiple sclerosis. Hum Mol Genet 18(4):767–778, doi:ddn388 [pii] 10.1093/hmg/ddn388

62. De Jager PL, Jia X, Wang J, de Bakker PI, Ottoboni L, Aggarwal NT, Piccio L, Raychaudhuri S, Tran D, Aubin C, Briskin R, Romano S, International MSGC, Baranzini SE, McCauley JL, Pericak-Vance MA, Haines JL, Gibson RA, Naeglin Y, Uitdehaag B, Matthews PM, Kappos L, Polman C, McArdle WL, Strachan DP, Evans D, Cross AH, Daly MJ, Compston A, Sawcer SJ, Weiner HL, Hauser SL, Hafler DA, Oksenberg JR (2009) Meta-analysis of genome scans and replication identify CD6, IRF8 and TNFRSF1A as new multiple sclerosis susceptibility loci. Nat Genet 41(7):776–782, doi:ng.401 [pii] 10.1038/ng.401

63. Australia, New Zealand Multiple Sclerosis Genetics Consortium (2009) Genome-wide association study identifies new multiple sclerosis susceptibility loci on chromosomes 12 and 20. Nat Genet 41(7):824–828. doi:10.1038/ng.396

64. Sanna S, Pitzalis M, Zoledziewska M, Zara I, Sidore C, Murru R, Whalen MB, Busonero F, Maschio A, Costa G, Melis MC, Deidda F, Poddie F, Morelli L, Farina G, Li Y, Dei M, Lai S, Mulas A, Cuccuru G, Porcu E, Liang L, Zavattari P, Moi L, Deriu E, Urru MF, Bajorek M, Satta MA, Cocco E, Ferrigno P, Sotgiu S, Pugliatti M, Traccis S, Angius A, Melis M, Rosati G, Abecasis GR, Uda M, Marrosu MG, Schlessinger D, Cucca F (2010) Variants within the immunoregulatory CBLB gene are associated with multiple sclerosis. Nat Genet 42(6):495–497. doi:10.1038/ng.584

65. Nischwitz S, Cepok S, Kroner A, Wolf C, Knop M, Muller-Sarnowski F, Pfister H, Roeske D, Rieckmann P, Hemmer B, Ising M, Uhr M, Bettecken T, Holsboer F, Muller-Myhsok B, Weber F (2010) Evidence for VAV2 and ZNF433 as susceptibility genes for multiple sclerosis. J Neuroimmunol 227(1–2):162–166. doi:10.1016/j.jneuroim.2010.06.003

66. Jakkula E, Leppa V, Sulonen AM, Varilo T, Kallio S, Kemppinen A, Purcell S, Koivisto K, Tienari P, Sumelahti ML, Elovaara I, Pirttila T, Reunanen M, Aromaa A, Oturai AB, Sondergaard HB, Harbo HF, Mero IL, Gabriel SB, Mirel DB, Hauser SL, Kappos L, Polman C, De Jager PL, Hafler DA, Daly MJ, Palotie A, Saarela J, Peltonen L (2010) Genome-wide association study in a high-risk isolate for multiple sclerosis reveals associated variants in STAT3 gene. Am J Hum Genet 86(2):285–291. doi:10.1016/j.ajhg.2010.01.017

67. Matesanz F, Gonzalez-Perez A, Lucas M, Sanna S, Gayan J, Urcelay E, Zara I, Pitzalis M, Cavanillas ML, Arroyo R, Zoledziewska M, Marrosu M, Fernandez O, Leyva L, Alcina A, Fedetz M, Moreno-Rey C, Velasco J, Real LM, Ruiz-Pena JL, Cucca F, Ruiz A, Izquierdo G (2012) Genome-wide association study of multiple sclerosis confirms a novel locus at 5p13.1. PLoS One 7(5):e36140. doi:10.1371/journal.pone.0036140

68. Martinelli-Boneschi F, Esposito F, Brambilla P, Lindstrom E, Lavorgna G, Stankovich J, Rodegher M, Capra R, Ghezzi A, Coniglio G, Colombo B, Sorosina M, Martinelli V, Booth D, Oturai AB, Stewart G, Harbo HF, Kilpatrick TJ, Hillert J, Rubio JP, Abderrahim H, Wojcik J, Comi G (2012) A genome-wide association study in progressive multiple sclerosis. Mult Scler 18(10):1384–1394. doi:10.1177/1352458512439118

69. Mastronardi FG, Noor A, Wood DD, Paton T, Moscarello MA (2007) Peptidyl argininedeiminase 2 CpG island in multiple sclerosis white matter is hypomethylated. J Neurosci Res 85(9):2006–2016. doi:10.1002/jnr.21329

70. D'Souza CA, Wood DD, She YM, Moscarello MA (2005) Autocatalytic cleavage of myelin basic protein: an alternative to molecular mimicry. Biochemistry 44(38):12905–12913. doi:10.1021/bi051152f

71. Makar KW, Wilson CB (2004) DNA methylation is a nonredundant repressor of the Th2 effector program. J Immunol 173(7):4402–4406

72. Akimzhanov AM, Yang XO, Dong C (2007) Chromatin remodeling of interleukin-17 (IL-17)-IL-17 F cytokine gene locus during inflammatory helper T cell differentiation. J Biol Chem 282(9):5969–5972. doi:10.1074/jbc.C600322200

73. Li H, He Y, Richardson WD, Casaccia P (2009) Two-tier transcriptional control of oligodendrocyte differentiation. Curr Opin Neurobiol 19(5):479–485. doi:10.1016/j.conb.2009.08.004

74. Mastronardi FG, Wood DD, Mei J, Raijmakers R, Tseveleki V, Dosch HM, Probert L, Casaccia-Bonnefil P, Moscarello MA (2006) Increased citrullination of histone H3 in multiple sclerosis brain and animal models of demyelination: a role for tumor necrosis factor-induced peptidylarginine deiminase 4 translocation. J Neurosci 26(44):11387–11396. doi:10.1523/JNEUROSCI.3349-06.2006

75. Tegla CA, Cudrici CD, Azimzadeh P, Singh AK, Trippe R 3rd, Khan A, Chen H, Andrian-Albescu M, Royal W 3rd, Bever C, Rus V, Rus H (2013) Dual role of response gene to complement-32 in multiple sclerosis. Exp Mol Pathol 94(1):17–28. doi:10.1016/j.yexmp.2012.09.005

76. Gao B, Kong Q, Kemp K, Zhao YS, Fang D (2012) Analysis of sirtuin 1 expression reveals a molecular explanation of IL-2-mediated reversal of T-cell tolerance. Proc Natl Acad Sci U S A 109(3):899–904. doi:10.1073/pnas.1118462109

77. Li K, Seo KH, Gao T, Zheng Q, Qi RQ, Wang H, Weiland M, Dong Z, Mi QS, Zhou L (2011) Invariant NKT cell development and function in microRNA-223 knockout mice. Int Immunopharmacol 11(5):561–568. doi:10.1016/j.intimp.2010.11.004

78. Junker A, Krumbholz M, Eisele S, Mohan H, Augstein F, Bittner R, Lassmann H, Wekerle H, Hohlfeld R, Meinl E (2009) MicroRNA profiling of multiple sclerosis lesions identifies modulators of the regulatory protein CD47. Brain 132(Pt 12):3342–3352. doi:10.1093/brain/awp300

79. Cox MB, Cairns MJ, Gandhi KS, Carroll AP, Moscovis S, Stewart GJ, Broadley S, Scott RJ, Booth DR, Lechner-Scott J, ANMSG Consortium (2010) MicroRNAs miR-17 and miR-20a inhibit T cell activation genes and are under-expressed in MS whole blood. PLoS One 5(8):e12132. doi:10.1371/journal.pone.0012132

INDEX

Barbara Stefanska and David J. MacEwan (eds.), *Epigenetics and Gene Expression in Cancer, Inflammatory and Immune Diseases*,
Methods in Pharmacology and Toxicology, DOI 10.1007/978-1-4939-6743-8, © Springer Science+Business Media LLC 2017

Printed in the United States
By Bookmasters